Conducting Case Studies in Remedial Massage Therapy

From Concept to Publication

Cover page by Jeremy Pluck

First published in 2025 in Australia by Publisher:
Pluck Pluck Goose
1 Vaucluse Crescent
Bellevue Heights 5050,
South Australia

ISBN 978-0-9756253-3-0

9 780975 625330

Foreword

This book is one of the most comprehensive you will ever read. It it's written in a language that we can all understand and in a way that takes us all through every step of the process of preparing for, writing and submitting, and publishing a case study and then giving back those benefits to all patients who have similar conditions through wider availability of our knowledge.

In a literal sense it leaves no stone unturned, every fact and every step will inform the novice investigator of what to do, how to do it and how to present, but will also inform the more experienced of the finer points of a good case study that we can sometimes forget about.

I hope that reading this will stimulate massage therapists and all others who have a unique piece of information about a unique individual and who have applied an appropriate treatment or management strategy to publish their findings to help lead to further investigations such as clinical trials to give improved outcomes to all those affected by the range of conditions a therapist can confidently treat.

We all very much need more information about how our treatments change outcomes and this book is a critical leverage point to help achieve that.

Congratulations to Andrea for her initiative in this process.

Professor Neil B Piller
Director Lymphoedema Clinical Research Unit
Flinders Centre for Innovation in Cancer
College of Medicine and Public Health
Flinders University, South Australia

Disclaimer

The content in this book is based on my personal experiences, professional knowledge, and research. It is intended for educational and informational purposes only and should not be considered medical, legal, or financial advice. While I strive to provide accurate and up-to-date information, I make no guarantees regarding the completeness, reliability, or applicability of the content to individual circumstances.

By engaging with this material, you acknowledge that I am not responsible for any outcomes—positive or negative—that may result from applying the concepts discussed. Your success depends on your unique situation, actions, and professional judgment.

If you have any concerns or require specific advice, please seek guidance from an appropriate expert.

Acknowledgements

This book represents my journey of passion, dedication, and a genuine belief in the power of case studies to elevate remedial massage therapy practice. I am incredibly grateful to all the massage therapists, educators, and health professionals who have inspired and supported me along the way.

A heartfelt thank you to my husband, Jeremy, whose support has been my anchor throughout this project. From helping me refine ideas to making our online course and this book more user-friendly and accessible, your patience, encouragement, and insights have been invaluable. I truly could not have done this without you.

To Leila S., my dear friend and editor, thank you for your unwavering support and keen eye for detail with this project. Your thoughtful suggestions and expert guidance have brought clarity and polish to this book, not to mention reduced the page numbers!

I am so grateful for the time and care you've invested. This book is all the better for your input. Thank you for being both a brilliant editor and an amazing friend.

Thank you, Neil P., for your valuable insights and suggestions, which helped refine this book. Your support is truly appreciated.

To my peers and mentors in the massage and lymphoedema communities, thank you for your wisdom, encouragement, and the knowledge you've so generously shared.

And to you—the massage therapist holding this book—thank you for your dedication to advancing our profession. Your willingness to learn, grow, and share your experiences through case studies is what keeps our industry moving forward.

Introduction

Welcome to *Case Studies in Massage Therapy: From Concept to Publication*. This book is here to guide you step-by-step through the process of creating, conducting, and presenting your own case study.

This book complements our online MassageCPE course at www.MassageCPE.com.au on conducting case studies, which you may have already completed or may wish to explore in the future. The course offers an interactive, step-by-step approach, while this book serves as a deeper dive and lasting reference guide. Whether you are exploring case studies for the first time or refining your approach, I have designed this resource to be practical, relatable, and easy to follow.

Case studies are so much more than academic exercises—they are stories. Stories of growth, discovery, and outcomes that can inspire others and improve the way we collaborate with our clients. When you share your observations, successes, and even challenges, you contribute to a valuable body of knowledge that benefits not just your practice, but our industry as a whole.

As you turn these pages, I hope you will find the confidence, and a sense of excitement for writing your own case study.

Contents

Case Studies

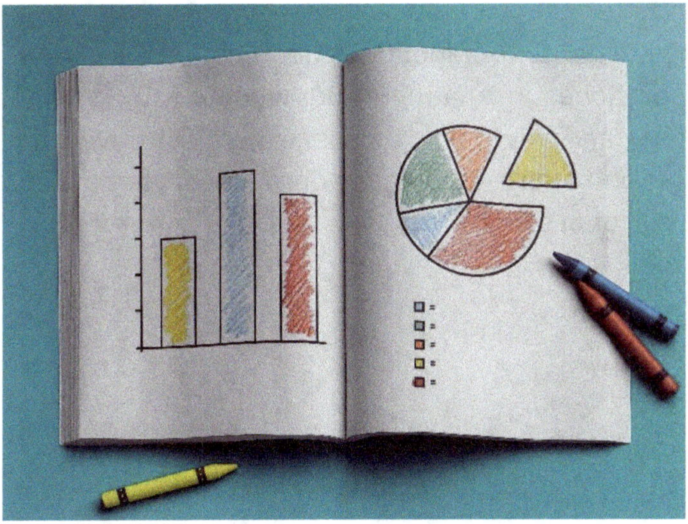

What are Case Studies?

A case study is an in-depth investigation of an individual client, treatment, or therapeutic intervention over a specific period. It captures the outcomes, the experience, challenges faced, adjustments made, and insights gained along the way.

Case studies are a cornerstone of evidence-informed practice in of any discipline. They provide an opportunity to document and share client experiences, therapeutic outcomes, and innovative approaches to treatment. But what exactly is a case study, and why should massage therapists invest their time and effort into creating one? I mean, Let's face it, it is a lot of extra work.

The Role of Case Studies

Case studies hold a unique and valuable place in massage therapy. They bridge the gap between hands-on practice and evidence-based research, offering a way for therapists to document their experiences, share their insights, and contribute to the broader professional community. While large-scale studies are often seen as the gold standard in research, case studies provide something equally important—a close-up look at real-world scenarios, client responses, and treatment outcomes.

They offer therapists a way to explore specific conditions, techniques, and client responses in detail, providing insights that generalised research might overlook.

One of the greatest strengths of a case study is its ability to tell a story. Behind every study is a person—a client with unique needs, challenges, and goals. By sharing these stories, we're not just presenting data; we're offering relatable, human-centered insights that can inspire and educate other therapists. Case studies remind us that every client is different, and every session has the potential to teach us something valuable.

They also provide a platform for innovation. Massage therapy is an evolving field, and therapists are often experimenting with new techniques, tools, and approaches to address complex client needs. A well-documented case study allows these creative problem-solving strategies to be shared and, in turn, refined by others.

Importantly, case studies help validate our work. They serve as tangible evidence of the effectiveness of our treatments, giving us the confidence to stand behind what we do. In a world where massage therapy is still fighting for recognition in some healthcare circles, every well-documented case study adds weight to our collective voice.

Finally, engaging in case study work isn't just about contributing to the profession—it's also a powerful tool for personal growth. The process encourages us to ask better questions, observe more closely, and reflect deeply on our practice. It challenges us to think critically and communicate clearly, skills that benefit not just our research but our day-to-day work with clients.

So, whether you're drawn to case studies for their storytelling potential, their ability to drive innovation, or their role in professional validation, know that your contribution makes a difference. Every case study adds a piece to the puzzle, helping to shape the future of massage therapy.

What You Can Expect from This Book

This book is a comprehensive guide to walk you step-by-step through the process of developing your own case study. It starts all aspects of the process from choosing a topic and gathering data to writing, presenting through to publishing your findings. Each chapter builds on the last to ensure you feel confident and capable.

Types of Case Studies

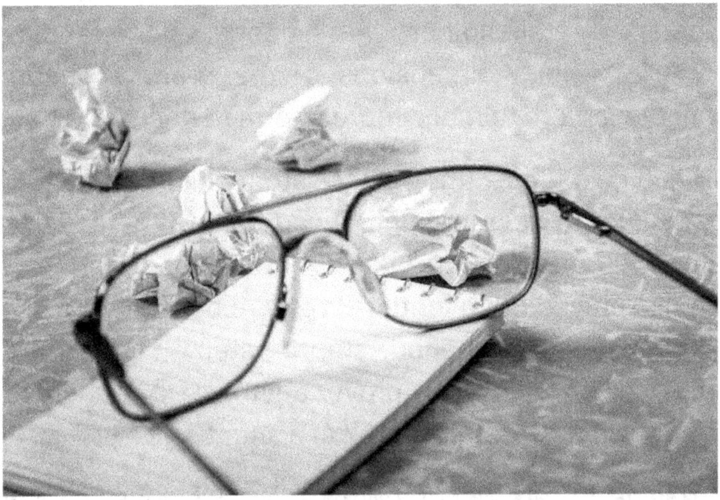

Photo by Steve

Descriptive Case Studies

Descriptive case studies focus on examining a specific event or issue to uncover key facts, explore what occurred, and identify the individuals or groups involved. They are often used to compare two instances of an event, highlighting their similarities and differences. Unlike other types of case studies, descriptive ones typically do not offer solutions or recommendations. Their primary goal is to provide readers or stakeholders with a deeper understanding of the various dimensions of the event or issue, enabling them to make more informed decisions.

This type of case study is the "storytelling" approach. It is about documenting the details of a specific client's condition, the treatment process, and how things played out over time. You are basically saying, "Here's what happened, step by step." You are not necessarily trying to prove anything, but instead offering a rich, detailed look at a situation.

Imagine you are working with a client who has ongoing back pain. You would start by describing their symptoms, what treatments you chose, and then you would document the changes over time—whether the pain decreased, what techniques worked best, and what adjustments were made. It is like a therapeutic journal, where the focus is all about capturing the journey.

Exploratory Case Studies

You will use an exploratory case study to investigate a topic or phenomenon in its early stages to develop a clearer understanding and identify key questions or areas for further research. The case study will focus on uncovering patterns and generating hypotheses, providing a foundation for more detailed and targeted studies. Rather than drawing definitive conclusions, an exploratory case study is designed to open avenues for deeper exploration and analysis.

If you are diving into something new or not well understood, an exploratory case study is where you want to be. It is more about exploring "what could happen" or "what's possible." You might not have all the answers yet, but you are experimenting, trying new approaches, and observing the outcomes.

For instance, you are trying a new massage technique on a client who has never responded well to traditional methods. You are exploring whether this new technique could be a game-changer. It is not about proving success, but more about asking questions, generating new ideas, and getting curious about what might be possible in the future.

Explanatory Case Studies

An explanatory case study will help you to explain *why* something worked or did not work. You are reporting facts as well as digging into the reasons behind those facts. You might look at the cause and effect: "Why did this treatment improve the client's condition?" or "What made this approach more effective than the last?"

For example, if a client with chronic neck tension found relief after a deep tissue session, you would take a deeper look at why that treatment worked for them. Was it the pressure? The technique? The timing of the session? This type of case study is where you start drawing connections and offering insights that others can use.

Intrinsic Case Studies

Intrinsic case studies are all about what makes a particular case special. This could be a unique client or a particularly complex situation. These cases usually stand out because there is something unusual about the client or the challenge they present.

As an example, let us say you have a client with a rare combination of issues (such as, lymphoedema and fibromyalgia). This case would be a good example of an intrinsic case study. In addition to documenting the symptoms and treatments, you are looking deeper into what makes this client's case unique, and how that uniqueness affects your treatment plan.

Instrumental Case Studies

An Instrumental case study focuses on a specific case to gain insight into a broader issue or phenomenon. The case itself is of secondary importance, serving primarily as a tool to understand, illustrate, or explore a larger concept or theory. This type of case study is particularly valuable when the chosen case provides a unique or illuminating perspective that enhances understanding of the wider subject matter.

It is a way to learn more about a bigger issue by examining one specific case. The goal here is not just to focus on the case, but to use it as a springboard for understanding a larger trend or question.

Suppose you are working with a client who has chronic shoulder pain, and you are trying a new combination of techniques. By focusing on this one case, you might learn something that could apply to a broader group of clients. The focus is less about the individual client and more about how that case helps you answer a bigger question, such as "What's the most effective way to treat chronic pain in the shoulder?"

Comparative Case Studies

As the name suggests, Comparative case studies are all about comparisons. If you are looking to see how different treatments or approaches work for similar conditions, this case study is a good way to do it. It gives you the opportunity to explore what works and what does not work, by looking at two or more cases side-by-side.

Say you are treating two clients with lower back pain—one with a sports injury and another with a sedentary lifestyle issue. You could compare how different massage techniques (for example, myofascial release versus Swedish) affect each client. This comparison helps you see how you can tailor treatments based on the individual's cause of pain.

Retrospective Case Studies

A Retrospective case study looks back at a case after the treatment is finished. It is like reflecting on a journey and analysing the results. You can assess the effectiveness of your interventions with the benefit of hindsight.

You might look back at a client you treated a year ago, someone who had severe muscle tension due to stress. Now that time has passed, you can assess whether the treatment you used really made a lasting impact. This kind of case study is about seeing how well the treatment “held up” over time and identifying areas for improvement or refinement.

Prospective Case Studies

You complete a Prospective case study when you need to identify a subject or group and observe them over time to study how specific factors influence outcomes. The approach of this case study is forward-looking with the focus on collecting data as events unfold rather than analysing past occurrences. They are particularly useful for 1. exploring cause-and-effect relationships, 2. tracking changes, 3. identifying trends, and 4. offering insights into dynamic processes as they occur.

Prospective case studies are all about following a client in real-time. You are tracking the treatment and results as they happen and observing and adjusting as you go.

Let’s say you have a new client with shoulder tightness. Over the course of a few weeks, you are documenting their response to different techniques, adjusting the plan based on their progress. This ongoing case study helps you make real-time decisions and track how treatment unfolds.

Single-Case Experimental Design (SCED)

SCED is a research method used to evaluate the effects of an intervention on a single subject or a small group of individuals. This approach is particularly common in fields like psychology, education, and healthcare.

SCED involves repeated measurements of a dependent variable – such as behaviour or symptom severity before, during, and after the introduction of an intervention. It uses this structured approach to observation to assess the relationship between the intervention and observed changes, often employing a baseline (A) and intervention (B) phase, such as in an A-B or A-B-A-B design.

The key strength of SCED is its ability to provide detailed, individualised insights into the effectiveness of an intervention while allowing for controlled comparisons within the same subject. It is especially valuable when larger-scale studies are impractical or when tailored interventions are required.

This is more of a scientific approach where you manipulate variables to see what has an effect. This is about actively testing out different treatment methods and using measurable data to see what works best.

If you are working with a client with knee pain, you might track their pain levels before and after using a certain technique, comparing results each time. You might adjust the pressure, timing, or even the frequency of sessions. This approach allows you to measure specific changes and document what makes the biggest difference in your client's outcomes.

These case study types offer a range of ways to look at your practice, from exploring new techniques to evaluating what is working with your current clients. Each type has its own strengths and depending on what you are trying to learn or share, one might suit you better than the others. Which one are you most drawn to when documenting your own cases?

Pros and Cons of Different Case Study Types

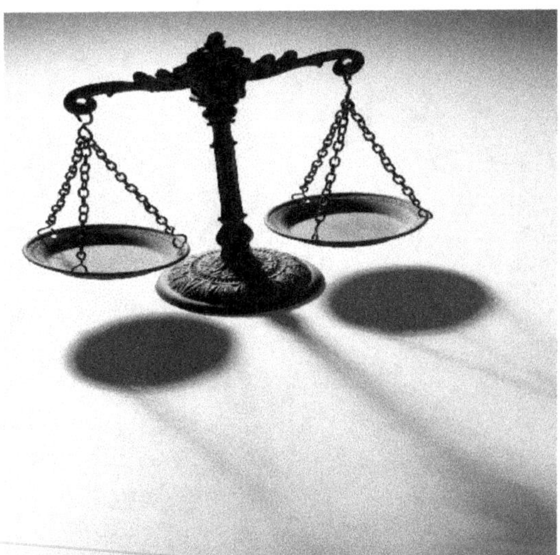

Now that we have explored the different types of case studies, let's have a closer look at some of their pros and cons. Understanding the strengths and limitations of each type can help you choose the right approach based on your goals and the case at hand.

Descriptive Case Studies

Pros

A Descriptive case study is relatively easy to write because it is primarily about telling a story, this is one of the simpler types of case studies to put together.

It gives you a well-rounded, comprehensive look at a client's journey, capturing the details of their treatment from start to finish.

If you are just starting to write case studies, this is a solid choice since it does not require a deep dive into theory or data analysis.

Cons

While detailed, a Descriptive case study does not always offer much in terms of lessons learned or broader takeaways. It is more of a snapshot than a thorough analysis because it provides limited insights.

Because Descriptive case studies focus on one individual, they lack generalisability. The findings might not apply to other clients with similar issues. It is not an ideal choice if you are looking for broader trends.

Exploratory Case Studies

Pros

Explorative case studies are great for uncovering new ideas. If you are venturing into uncharted territory or trying something new, you can obtain valuable insights which can help you think outside the box for possible client treatments.

They can help to generate curiosity and open the door for new questions and possibilities, which can lead to further exploration and research.

Cons

Exploratory case studies are less definitive. Because you are exploring new ground, you might not reach clear conclusions right away, making it harder to draw concrete lessons.

They also require more observation. You may need to conduct multiple cases or follow up over time to really understand the full impact of your approach.

Explanatory Case Studies

Pros

This type of case study helps you get to the "why" behind what works and what does not, giving you a deeper understanding of your treatment methods.

By focusing on cause and effect, you will gain insights that can improve your approach and decision-making in future treatments, helping you to refine your practice.

If you are trying to establish why a certain technique is effective, this is an excellent choice.

Cons

Explanatory case studies can be complex. You will need to dig deeper into theory and data, which can be time-consuming and require a more detailed analysis.

To make solid conclusions, you may need to ensure other variables are controlled, and controlled conditions can be tricky in the real-world therapy setting.

Intrinsic Case Studies

Pros

If you have got a particularly rare or interesting case, this type of study can shed light on something that has not been explored much, making it valuable to the community.

These cases are often more compelling because they are unusual or unique, which can make the case study more interesting for readers.

Cons

Since you are focusing on a unique case, it can be harder to apply the findings to other clients.

If the case is highly specific, others may not be able to replicate the treatment for similar results.

Instrumental Case Studies

Pros

Even though you are focusing on one case, the insights you gain can often be applied to other situations, making this a great choice for drawing broader conclusions.

Instrumental case studies are helpful for understanding big questions. If you are tackling a larger issue, like the effectiveness of a new technique, this case can serve as a model for exploring similar cases.

Cons

While it helps answer broader questions, you are still working with a particular case. It might not be enough to draw strong, wide-reaching conclusions on its own.

You will need to connect the dots between your specific case and the bigger issue you are studying, which may involve more time and research.

Comparative Case Studies

Pros

Comparative case studies highlight differences and patterns. They allow you to directly compare how different treatments work for similar issues, which can help you fine-tune your approach.

They are very useful for developing effective strategies, as you get to see what works and what doesn't when it comes to real clients and their conditions.

Cons

To do it right, you need at least two cases to compare. That means more time and effort on your part, especially if you need to track multiple clients over time.

Every client is different, so it might be difficult to ensure that the treatments are comparable enough to make valid conclusions. It can be a real challenge to control variables.

Retrospective Case Studies

Pros

Retrospective case studies are easier to analyse. Since you are looking back on completed treatments, you can draw from actual results and reflect on what worked best.

This type allows you to evaluate how well your interventions worked in real-life scenarios and identify areas for improvement, which is useful to refine your practice.

Cons

You do not have the luxury of adjusting things as you go since the treatment has already happened.

Looking back at a case might lead to hindsight bias, where you believe you saw success in an area that was not hugely significant.

Prospective Case Studies

Pros

Following a client through their treatment allows you to track progress as it happens, giving you fresh insights that can be immediately applied.

Since you are actively treating the client, you can tweak the treatment plan if something is not working and observe the effects in real time.

Cons

Prospective case studies are time-consuming. Tracking a client over weeks or months requires dedication, and results may not be immediately clear.

You will need to document each session and any changes in the treatment plan, which can add to your workload.

Single-Case Experimental Design (SCED)

Pros

SCEDs are highly structured and data driven. This type is great if you want to test specific hypotheses or techniques with measurable outcomes.

By isolating variables and focusing on one client, you can better understand what works and why.

Cons

To be effective, you need to have a clear hypothesis and structured approach, which takes time to set up.

Because SCED is so focused on control and measurement, it may not always reflect the messy, dynamic nature of real-world treatments.

Each of these case study types offers its own advantages, but they also come with challenges. It is all about finding the right fit for the information you are trying to uncover and the type of client you are working with. Depending on your goals, you might even find that combining several types of case studies works best.

Which type of case study do you feel most drawn to for your practice or writing?

Take some time now and write down the one(s) that appeal to you.

Page left intentionally blank for your notes.

Ethical Considerations

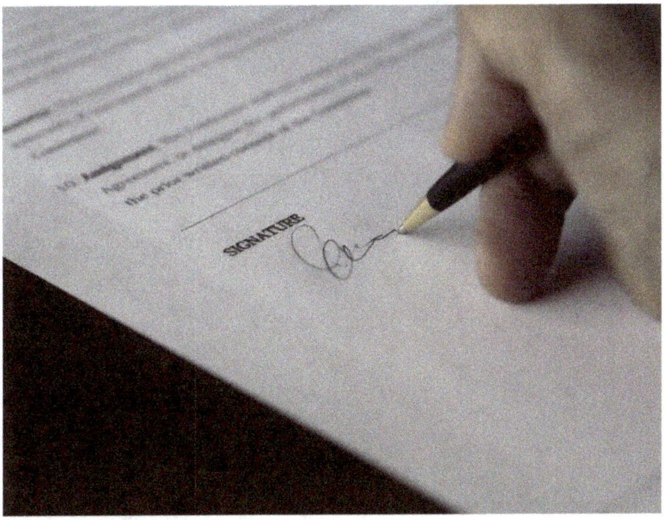

The key ethical principles in conducting case studies form the foundation in which professionalism, trust, and respect is maintained for all the individuals involved. This section outlines what each principle means in practice and how it applies to conducting ethical case studies.

Informed Consent

Informed consent is non-negotiable. Before you document or share any details about a client's case, you need to ensure they understand exactly what you are doing and give you explicit permission. Informed consent means explaining to the client how their information will be used, ensuring they understand the potential outcomes, and letting them know they have the right to withdraw consent at any time.

Informed consent is a legal requirement in most places, and it is about respecting your client's autonomy and ensuring they are fully aware of what is going on. For example, if you are using their case in a published study, a class, or even just as a learning tool, they need to agree to it.

You can create a simple consent form that outlines how their case will be used, what kind of information will be shared (in what context), and who will see it. Keep the language clear, and make sure the client has time to ask questions.

Confidentiality and Privacy

One of the core ethical principles in any healthcare setting is maintaining confidentiality. In the context of case studies, this means ensuring that any personal identifying information about your client (like their full name, contact details, or specific medical history) is kept private.

Respecting confidentiality builds trust with your clients and ensures they feel safe sharing sensitive information. It is also legally required in Australia under laws like the Privacy Act 1988, Australian Privacy Principals, My Health Records Act 2012, and other State and Territory Legislations. There are similar regulations in other countries.

When writing a case study, remove any identifiable details from the case, such as full names or contact information. You can either anonymise the data or get explicit permission to use the information with the client's name. In many cases, it is important to change certain details (like age, occupation, or geographic location) to protect privacy.

Accuracy and Honesty

Ethical case studies should present an accurate and honest account of the situation. You need to document the challenges and successes, not just the ones that support your original hypothesis.

Inaccurate reporting can mislead other practitioners and even harm clients if others base their decisions on your findings. Plus, honesty is essential to building credibility in your work.

Document everything truthfully, including both the successes and the setbacks. You can also document the struggles because those often provide valuable learning opportunities for others.

Respect for Client Autonomy

Even if a client agrees to take part in a case study, their autonomy should be respected throughout the process. You need to allow the client to make decisions about their involvement and not pressure them into participating.

Clients should feel empowered in the decision-making process, knowing that they can opt out at any time without any negative repercussions to their treatment. Their comfort with the process should always come first.

You should let your client know they have the freedom to withdraw their consent at any time, and make sure they understand there is no impact on their treatment or relationship with you. Keep communication open and check in with them regularly about their comfort level.

Beneficence (Do No Harm)

This is a principle we are all familiar with—always act in the best interests of your clients. In the context of case studies, this means ensuring that taking part in the case study will not negatively affect your client's care or well-being in any way.

The main priority is always your client's health and safety. Conducting case studies should not interfere with the quality of care or cause harm to your client.

Make sure that the treatments or interventions you are testing do not pose unnecessary risks, and that all case study activities are secondary to the client's primary care and well-being.

Cultural Sensitivity

Every client comes from a different background, and it is important that you respect their cultural beliefs and practices when conducting case studies. This means understanding and respecting their values and preferences as part of your documentation.

Cultural sensitivity ensures that you are treating your clients with respect and not imposing any beliefs or practices that might be foreign or uncomfortable to them. It also broadens your understanding, helping you become a more holistic practitioner.

Engage in open and respectful conversations with your clients about their preferences, beliefs, and any cultural factors that might influence their treatment or participation in a case study. Acknowledge these aspects in your case documentation when relevant, ensuring that you do not make assumptions or generalise.

Use of Client Data

The use of client data in case studies is sensitive. It is vital that you make sure that any data used—whether it is treatment details, outcomes, or personal history—stays secure and is used appropriately.

Client data is personal and should be handled with the utmost care. Misuse or mishandling of data can lead to legal and ethical issues, and it can harm the trust you have worked so hard to build with your clients.

Store client information securely, whether it is digital or paper. If you plan to use any data in a case study, get explicit consent, and ensure that the data is anonymised as much as possible. Be clear about how and where the data will be used, and ensure it is only shared with people who have a legitimate need to know.

Publication and Dissemination

If you plan to publish your case study, you need to carefully consider how you present your findings. Will it be shared in a journal? Will you include it in a training session? Whatever the method, always be mindful of how the information is communicated to others.

Ethical publishing ensures that the findings you share are accurate, relevant, and do not mislead the reader. It also means giving credit where it is due and not plagiarising other people's work or ideas.

Be transparent about how you collected the data, what conclusions you are drawing, and the limitations of your study. If you are referencing other sources, cite them properly, and make sure you have permission if needed.

These ethical considerations are all about balancing the need for knowledge and growth with the responsibility we have to our clients. By staying mindful of these principles, you ensure that your case studies are both valuable and respectful of those you work with. How do these considerations resonate with you in your practice?

Challenges and Limitations of Case Studies

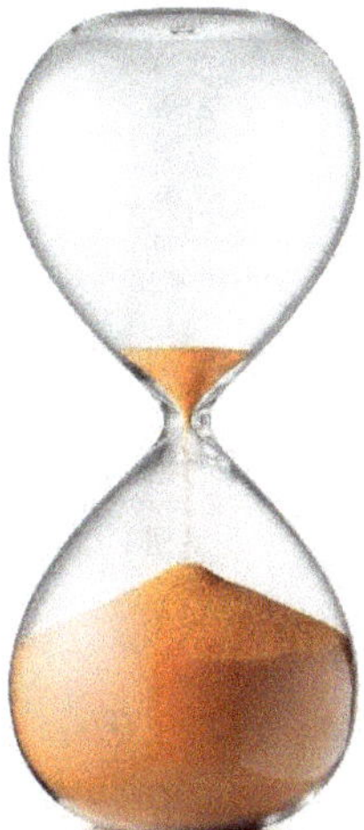

When conducting case studies, you are bound to run into a few bumps along the way—some of which might test your patience, creativity, and adaptability. But that is all part of the learning process! Let's talk about some of the ~~most~~ common challenges and limitations you might face and how to handle them.

Small Sample Size

In case studies, you are usually working with one (or a few) clients at a time, which means your sample size is limited. This is different from larger-scale research where you might have hundreds of participants to draw from. The smaller sample size can make it harder to generalise your findings to the broader population.

While a case study can offer in-depth insights into a specific client or scenario, it does not necessarily mean the same conclusions apply to all clients or situations. This can be frustrating if you are hoping to draw broader conclusions or convince others that your findings are universally applicable.

Be transparent about the limitations of your case study. Acknowledge that your findings are specific to the individual you worked with and might not translate directly to everyone. You can still draw valuable conclusions, but make sure to frame them carefully. You could also consider a series of case studies to build a broader base of evidence over time.

Subjectivity and Bias

Because you are the researcher and therapist, your own perspectives, assumptions, and experiences can influence the way you interpret the data and the results. This is known as researcher bias, and it is something every case study is at risk of.

If you are not careful, personal bias can skew the results of your case study, making them less objective. For example, if you have a preferred treatment method or approach, you might inadvertently focus only on outcomes that align with your expectations, overlooking other factors that do not fit.

Stay as neutral and objective as possible when gathering data and interpreting results. One strategy is to involve a second party—a colleague, mentor, or peer—who can review your findings and provide feedback. Keeping detailed and accurate records can also help minimise the impact of bias, making sure your conclusions are grounded in the data rather than your preferences.

Time and Resource Constraints

Case studies can be time-consuming. Between client sessions, data collection, documentation, and analysis, you might find yourself spending more time than you expected. Plus, there are logistical challenges like scheduling sessions and finding the time to gather all the data you need.

The time commitment can limit the depth and scope of your study. You may have to make compromises in terms of how thorough you can be, especially if you are working on the case study alongside your regular work or other professional responsibilities.

It is important to plan ahead and set realistic expectations for what you can achieve within your available time. Break the case study into smaller tasks and then allocate specific time slots for each step. If you are finding it hard to balance the workload, consider simplifying the study's scope to focus on a smaller question or outcome. You could also consider outsourcing certain aspects of the research process, like data analysis, if you need extra support.

Limited Control Over Variables

In a case study, you are dealing with real people, real conditions, and real complexities. Unlike controlled research environments, you cannot always control every variable that might influence the outcome. This can include things like the client's personal circumstances, external factors (for example, stressors at home), or even their commitment to the treatment plan.

The lack of control over these variables makes it harder to pinpoint exactly which factors led to a particular outcome. For example, if a client's progress is slower than expected, it might be due to their lifestyle, external stressors, or something unrelated to your treatment. This complicates the ability to draw clear conclusions.

Document all potential variables and influences as part of your case study. This might mean asking your client about lifestyle factors or tracking any changes in their environment that could affect their progress. Being transparent about these factors in your final analysis will help you present a more accurate picture and avoid over-generalising your findings.

Ethical Dilemmas

As mentioned earlier, ethical issues are always a concern in case studies, especially when it comes to obtaining informed consent, ensuring confidentiality, and balancing the needs of your client with the demands of your research. Navigating these issues can sometimes be tricky, particularly if there are unexpected challenges along the way.

Ethical concerns can jeopardise the integrity of your study, as well as the trust your clients place in you. Failing to address these issues appropriately could lead you to legal complications or damage your professional reputation.

Always adhere to ethical guidelines, and do not cut corners. If you are unsure about a particular ethical issue, consult with someone who can provide guidance. Regularly check in with your client to ensure they are comfortable with how the case study is progressing and make adjustments as needed. Transparency and honesty are key for you to maintain ethical integrity throughout the process.

Data Collection and Analysis Challenges

Gathering and interpreting data in a case study can be tricky. Whether you are relying on subjective measures like client feedback or objective data such as physical assessments, it can sometimes be difficult to make sense of what the data is telling you. The analysis of the data requires careful consideration to avoid misinterpretation.

It is important to collect and analyse data properly, or else you might miss key insights or make erroneous conclusions. Misinterpreting data can also lead to ineffective treatment plans or missed opportunities for improving client care.

Use a systematic approach to data collection and analysis. Keep your data organised and ensure you are consistently applying the same methods throughout the study. Consider using established tools or frameworks for analysing your data, and if needed, seek out additional resources (such as books, articles, or colleagues) to guide your analysis.

Unforeseen Client Outcomes

Sometimes, despite your best efforts, the outcome of a case study does not go as expected. Your client might not show the progress you hoped for, or the treatment plan might not have the intended results.

Unexpected outcomes can be discouraging and make it difficult to draw meaningful conclusions. It may also lead to feelings of frustration or disappointment, both for you and for your client.

Take a step back and reassess the situation. Sometimes, the case study process reveals more questions than answers, and that is okay. Document everything carefully, including why you think the results were different than expected, and use this as an opportunity to refine your methods or treatment strategies.

Even unexpected outcomes can provide valuable learning experiences that can guide future practices.

Time Constraints for Documentation

Case studies require careful, detailed documentation throughout the process, but finding the time to document everything thoroughly can be a challenge. As therapists, we often focus on the client's immediate needs and may overlook the importance of recording every detail in real-time.

Incomplete or rushed documentation can lead to inaccuracies and missed details, which can compromise the quality and validity of your case study. This can also impact the value of your study if others need to refer back to your records.

Make documentation part of your routine and try to fill in details immediately after each session rather than leaving it to the end. You should set aside specific time for reflection and note-taking, so you do not fall behind. It is also helpful to use digital tools or templates to streamline the process and ensure consistency.

Every case study will have its challenges, but they are all part of the process that helps you grow as a practitioner and researcher. Embrace the obstacles as opportunities for learning and refining your methods. When you acknowledge these limitations and plan for them, you can navigate them more effectively and ultimately create stronger, more insightful case studies.

Preparing for a Case study

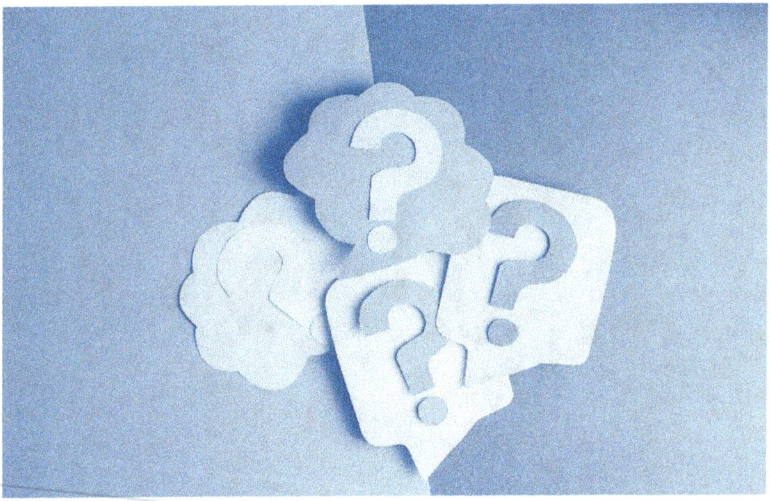

The foundation of every successful case study begins with selecting the right topic. Your topic will guide your research, shape your observations, and ultimately determine the impact of your work. In this chapter, we will explore how to identify a meaningful and relevant topic that aligns with your interests, expertise, and the needs of the massage therapy community.

Factors to Consider When Selecting a Topic

A well-chosen topic ensures that your case study remains focused, engaging, and valuable to both you and your audience. It should address a specific question, challenge, or observation that contributes to the broader field of massage therapy.

Ask yourself if the topic is relevant. Does the topic address a current issue or knowledge gap in massage therapy?

Also think about feasibility. Do you have access to the resources, clients, and time needed to conduct the study?

And what about impact? Will the findings of your study offer meaningful insights or improvements to practice?

Brainstorm Your Topic

Choosing a meaningful topic starts with reflection and curiosity. Take some time to think about your experiences in practice. Have you noticed recurring challenges or patterns with your clients? Are there specific techniques or approaches you are drawn to and want to explore further?

Sometimes, the best ideas come from those "I wonder why" or "What if" moments during a treatment session. You might also recall interesting or unexpected outcomes from your work that sparked curiosity. Don't be afraid to think big at this stage. The goal is to generate as many ideas as possible without worrying about whether they are perfect or refined.

Write down your thoughts, questions, or even observations from your practice. This initial brainstorming phase is about letting your curiosity guide you to help identify potential areas of focus.

Take some time to reflect on your practice and experiences and ask yourself:

What recurring challenges do I notice with my clients?

Are there treatment techniques or approaches I would like to explore more deeply?

Have I observed interesting or unexpected outcomes in my sessions?

Choosing the Right Publication for Your Case Study

When selecting a topic for your case study, it is essential to consider where you would like to publish it and the specific requirements of your chosen journal. Many major lymphology journals for example, have strict guidelines, and failing to meet their criteria could mean that even a well-conducted case study is not accepted for publication.

There are now journals dedicated exclusively to case studies, which can be a valuable option. However, the downside is that these journals often have a smaller readership within the specific field of expertise, which may impact visibility. That said, with modern search tools and indexing systems, access to published work is broader than ever.

If the goal of publishing the case study includes professional promotion or career advancement, it's important to not only find a relevant journal but also consider its impact factor. A high-impact journal increases the study's credibility and reach, making it more influential within the field.

Refine Your Topic

Once you have gathered some initial ideas, it's time to narrow your focus and define your topic more clearly. A broad topic like "The effects of massage therapy on post-surgery recovery" can be refined into something more specific, such as "The effects of dynamic silicone cupping on scar tissue mobility after surgery."

Refining your topic helps ensure your study remains manageable and focused, which in turn allows you to dive deeper into a specific question rather than skimming the surface of a broad issue.

As you refine, ask yourself whether your topic is realistic given your resources, time, and access to clients. Does it address a meaningful question? Will it provide insights that are valuable to both you and the wider massage therapy community? Taking the time to sharpen your topic at this stage will set a solid foundation for the rest of your case study journey.

You should now have a clear, well-defined topic that serves as a solid foundation for your case study. Take your time with this step—it is one of the most important parts of the process. Write your ideas on the next page.

Page left intentionally blank for your notes

Defining Objectives and Goals

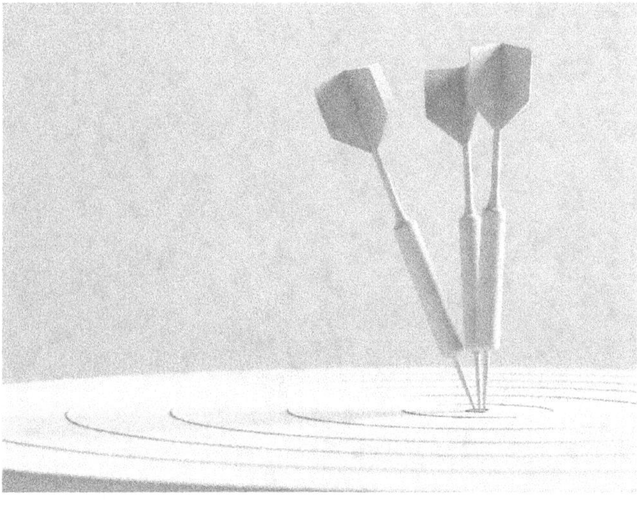

Setting clear objectives and goals is like having a roadmap for your case study journey. Without them, it is easy to get off track, or worse, end up somewhere completely unexpected. But when you take the time to define these from the start, it gives you a sense of direction and purpose, ensuring that every step you take is moving you toward the outcome you want.

Build a Strong Foundation with Objectives and Goals

Objectives and goals are your guiding stars before you even begin conducting your case study. They keep you grounded and focused, no matter what twists and turns you encounter along the way.

Build a strong foundation as follows:

- **Focus and Clarity** - Clear objectives help you narrow down what you are trying to achieve. They ensure that your research and treatment plans are aligned with a specific purpose, preventing you from getting bogged down in unnecessary details.

- **Measurable Outcomes** - Well-defined goals give you something concrete to measure. Without them, it can be difficult to assess progress or determine whether your case study has been successful.

- **Accountability** - Having specific objectives and goals means you are setting clear expectations—not just for yourself, but for your clients too. This helps manage expectations and ensures everyone is on the same page.

- **Guidance for Analysis** - With objectives in mind, you will know exactly what to look for in your data. Whether you are analysing physical outcomes, client feedback, or treatment responses, your goals will direct your attention to the most valuable information.

Set SMART Goals

You can set effective goals is by using the SMART framework. SMART stands for Specific, Measurable, Achievable, Relevant, and Time-bound, outlined as follows:

- **Specific** - Your goals should be clear and well-defined. Instead of saying, "I want to improve my client's well-being," a more specific goal would be, "I want to reduce my client's lower back pain by 30 percent within six weeks."

- **Measurable** - Make sure you can track progress and determine success. Using the "Specific" example above , you could measure pain reduction through regular pain assessments (for example, 1–10 scale) and compare them at the end of each week.

- **Achievable** - Set goals that are realistic given your resources, time, and the complexity of the case. If your client has a chronic condition, do not aim for a complete cure within a short time; instead, focus on improving symptoms or function gradually.

- **Relevant** - Your goal should align with the purpose of the case study and the needs of your client. For example, if your client's main concern is improving range of motion in their shoulder, setting a goal related to reducing stress might not be as relevant.

- **Time-bound** - Establish a time frame for achieving your goal – for example, "I aim to reduce my client's pain by 30 percent within six weeks" sets a clear timeline for assessing progress.

Example of Defining Objectives and Goals

Let's take a look at an example of how you might set objectives and goals for a case study:

Objective

To evaluate the effectiveness of a specific therapeutic technique (for example, deep tissue massage) in managing chronic neck pain for a client who has been experiencing discomfort for over a year.

Goals

1. Reduce neck pain by 25 percent (measured using a pain scale) within four weeks of treatment.
2. Increase the client's neck mobility by 10 percent (measured through range of motion tests) by the end of four weeks.
3. Enhance the client's overall satisfaction with treatment, aiming for at least an 80 percent satisfaction rate on a post-treatment survey.

With these objectives and goals in mind, you will have a clear direction for your case study. You will know exactly what data to collect, how to measure your client's progress, and when you can evaluate the results.

Align Your Case Study with Client Goals

Remember, your client's goals and needs should always be at the heart of your case study. If your client's priority is managing pain but they also want to feel more relaxed or have improved sleep quality, these goals should be factored into your objectives.

Example of Client-Centred Goals

- **Client Goal**: "I want to reduce pain in my shoulders and neck."
    - **Objective**: To reduce pain and discomfort in the neck and shoulders through massage therapy.
    - **Goal**: Reduce pain levels by 30 percent over the next six weeks, measured by the client's self-reported pain scale at the start and end of each session.
- **Client Goal**: "I want to improve my ability to move without feeling stiff."
    - **Objective**: To increase range of motion and flexibility through targeted techniques.

- **Goal**: Increase neck rotation by 15 degrees over eight weeks, measured using physical assessments.

Flexibility is Key

While it is essential to set clear objectives and goals, it is equally important to remain flexible. Case studies often evolve as new information comes to light or when circumstances change. Being open to adjusting your goals or methods along the way allows you to tailor your approach to best meet the client's needs.

Setting clear objectives and goals for your case study ensures that you are not only gathering relevant data but that you are also evaluating outcomes in a meaningful way. With SMART goals and client-centered objectives, you will have the clarity and structure you need to make your case study a success. Plus, by regularly checking in on your goals, you can adjust as needed to keep things on track—and that is what makes case studies so valuable for growth and learning!

Define YOUR Objectives and Goals

At this point it is time to lay the groundwork. Grab a notebook, your laptop, or whatever you like to write on. This book has some intentionally left blank pages so you can write some notes.

1. **Define Your Why:** Write down *why* you want to do this case study. Is it to explore a specific massage technique? To track a client's long-term progress? To contribute to the field?
2. **Set Your Goals:** Now, jot down three clear goals for your case study. Remember the SMART rule – Specific, Measurable, Achievable, Relevant, and Time-bound.
3. **Check for Alignment:** Take a moment to ask yourself: *Do my goals align with my 'why'?* If not, tweak them until they feel right.

If this case study goes exactly as planned, what is the one insight you hope to walk away with?

Page left intentionally blank for your notes.

Gathering Initial Data for your Case Study

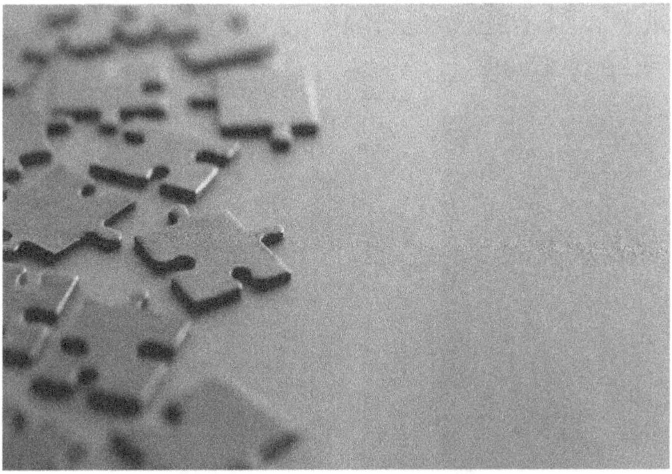

Before you jump into treatment or any interventions, it is essential to gather initial data that helps you understand your client's starting point. This data forms the foundation of your case study and allows you to track progress, measure outcomes, and make informed decisions as you go along. Without this step, it is like trying to navigate without a map—you will likely end up lost!

Let's walk through some key steps to gather initial data effectively.

Initial Client Assessment

This is where the case study begins! The initial assessment is an in-depth process that helps you understand your client's needs, concerns, and goals. You will gather personal and medical information, as well as a detailed history of their condition or symptoms.

Interview the Client

Ask about their lifestyle, history of symptoms, current complaints, and what they hope to achieve from the treatment. This will give you a clear idea of their expectations and help you set realistic goals for your case study.

Ask About Relevant Medical History

Gather information about any pre-existing conditions, medications, surgeries, or injuries that could impact the treatment plan. This helps you identify potential red flags or contraindications.

Clarify Client Goals

Make sure you fully understand what your client wants to achieve. This might include reducing pain, improving flexibility, or something more specific, like preparing for a specific physical challenge.

The initial assessment sets the tone for everything else in your case study. The more thorough and honest your client is, the better your understanding of their needs will be. This information also ensures that you are creating a treatment plan that is realistic and safe.

Physical Evaluation

The physical evaluation is your opportunity to get hands-on with your client and assess their current physical condition. This is where you can measure things like range of motion, muscle tension, pain levels, posture, and more.

Perform Range of Motion (ROM) Tests

Depending on your client's condition, assessing their ROM can help you see where they are limited and track improvements over time.

Conduct Posture Analysis

Check their posture, alignment, and any imbalances. Postural issues can often be tied to chronic pain or discomfort, so it is crucial to note any deviations from the norm.

Palpation for Muscle Tension or Trigger Points

If your client is experiencing pain, palpating the muscles to identify areas of tension or trigger points can be incredibly helpful. This will guide your treatment strategies and let you monitor changes in muscle tightness over time.

Pain Assessment

Use a consistent scale to assess pain levels (like the 0–10 scale). This is important for tracking changes in pain over the course of your treatment.

Functional Movement Screen

If relevant to your client's goals, a basic functional movement screen can help you assess their ability to perform certain tasks or movements (for example, squatting, bending).

This physical evaluation helps you understand the specifics of what your client is dealing with. It provides baseline measurements, so when you start treatment, you can track improvements or setbacks. Plus, it helps you tailor the treatment to your client's unique needs and challenges.

Client Feedback and Observations

You will also want to gather qualitative data through your client's own observations and experiences. These might not be as easily measured as physical assessments, but they are just as important for understanding the broader impact of the condition on their life.

Subjective Symptoms

Ask your client about how they are feeling—emotionally, mentally, and physically. Are they experiencing fatigue, stress, or sleep disruptions related to their condition? These factors can influence treatment and recovery.

Pain Journals

Encourage your client to keep a pain or symptom journal. This can help track daily fluctuations in pain, mobility, or mood and provide additional insight into how their condition is affecting their daily life.

It is always preferable to use previously validated tools for what ever the focus of the study is, for example Quality of Life or Pain scales - the addition and consideration of these validated tools adds strength and weight to the study.

Functional Impact
Have your client describe how their condition impacts their daily activities. Can they walk without pain? Are they limited in work or leisure activities? These insights give you a more holistic view of their situation.

Client feedback gives you a deeper understanding of how their condition is affecting their life outside of your therapy room. It also helps you evaluate the emotional and psychological aspects of their condition, which can be just as important as the physical ones.

Baseline Measurements

Once you have done the assessment and physical evaluation, it is time to establish measurable baselines for your study. These are your starting points for tracking progress over time.

Quantify Pain and Function

Use standardised tools to assess pain, flexibility, strength, and any other relevant metrics. For example, you could use the Visual Analog Scale (VAS) to measure pain levels, or a goniometer to measure joint mobility.

Document All Findings

Make sure to write down all baseline measurements in a detailed, organised manner. These will serve as a reference point for later comparisons, so accuracy is key.

Track External Factors

Sometimes, external factors like sleep quality, diet, or stress levels can influence a client's condition. Track these factors if they are relevant to your case study.

Baseline measurements allow you to track your client's progress and assess the effectiveness of your treatment. Without these data points, it would be difficult to measure the extent of improvement.

Although you need to track external factors, through interaction with the participant ask them to also try to minimise them so your study has less external confounders or they are small in impact.

Create a Treatment Plan Outline

At this stage, you should have enough information to start formulating a treatment plan. Based on the initial data, you can decide on the best therapeutic approaches and how to monitor their progress as follows:

- **Set Realistic Goals** - Based on the initial data, ensure your treatment goals are achievable and aligned with your client's expectations.

- **Tailor Treatment Approaches** - Use the information you have gathered to design a treatment plan that addresses the specific needs of your client. Consider using techniques that target their particular pain points or areas of limitation.

- **Establish Milestones** - Break down your treatment goals into smaller, measurable milestones. These milestones can serve as checkpoints for you and your client to track progress.

Your treatment plan is the roadmap to achieving the goals you have set for the case study. It is the strategy that will guide your interventions, and having a clear plan based on initial data will increase the chances of success.

Gathering initial data is the foundation of a successful case study. It provides the critical baseline you need to measure progress, tailor your treatment, and ensure you are addressing all aspects of your client's condition. By conducting a thorough assessment, physical evaluation, and gathering feedback, you are setting yourself up to not only understand your client's situation better but also to track and document meaningful change throughout the process.

Now that you have all this initial information, you will be able to make data-driven decisions as you move forward with your case study, ensuring that every step you take is supported by solid evidence.

Sometimes the data can be disappointing or not useful so don't be afraid of changing or deleting or adding to the data sets collected at any time - this matters for a normal research study but not a case study and in fact can be part of its development.

Exercise

1. **Create Your Data Checklist:** Write down all the information you will need from your client – health history, current symptoms, treatment goals, baseline assessments, etc.

2. **Choose Your Tools:** Decide how you will gather this data – will you use intake forms, interviews, physical assessments, or a mix of these?

3. **Plan Your First Meeting:** Draft a few key questions you will ask during your initial consultation.

How will you make sure your client feels comfortable sharing this information with you?

Page left intentionally blank for your notes.

Designing The Case Study

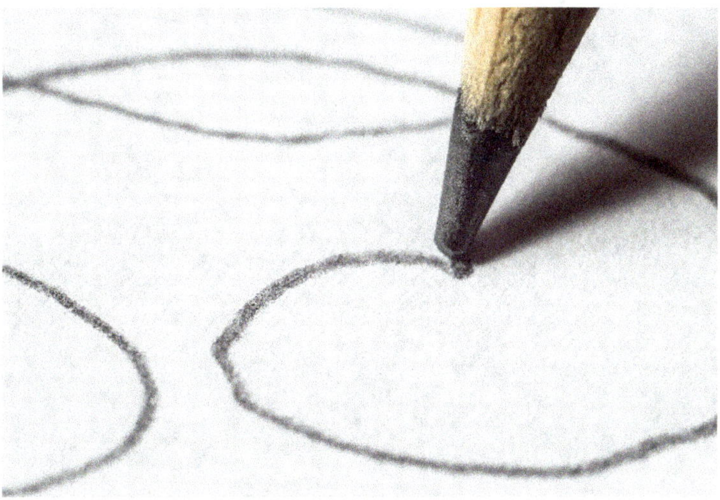

Designing a case study involves outlining how you will collect and analyse data, decide on your treatment approach, and structure your report. Your goal is to ensure that the study is clear, focused, and effective in demonstrating the value of your interventions.

Define the Scope and Focus

Before you even start designing the specifics of your case study, it is essential to clearly define the focus of the case study.

Defining the scope gives your case study sets a clear direction. It also helps you maintain focus, ensuring that you are not trying to solve everything at once. The clearer your focus, the easier it will be to measure success.

Define the scope and focus as follows:

- **Clarify the Problem** - It is important to identify the primary issue you are addressing with your client – for example, is it chronic pain, range of motion issues, post-surgical recovery, or something else?

- **Set Boundaries** - Be specific about what aspects of the client's condition or treatment you will focus on. For example, you might decide to focus solely on improving range of motion, or you may be addressing multiple issues like pain relief and stress reduction.

- **Establish Treatment Focus** - Choose the therapeutic methods you will apply. Are you using massage, myofascial release, trigger point therapy, or something else? Define which techniques and approaches you will be using in the study.

Choose Your Methodology

It is worth noting that **Method** refers to the specific techniques, procedures, or tools used to collect and analyse data in a study—for example, surveys, interviews, or clinical assessments. It's the *how* of conducting research. **Methodology**, on the other hand, is the overarching framework or philosophy that guides the choice and application of methods. It explains the *why* behind selecting certain methods and how they fit within a broader research approach, such as qualitative, quantitative, or mixed methods. In short, methods are the practical steps, while methodology is the theoretical justification behind those steps.

At this point determine how you will collect data and track your client's progress throughout the study. It is necessary to have a structured approach for gathering and evaluating information.

Having a clear methodology ensures that your data is consistent and comparable. Without a structured approach, you can easily become lost in the details or you may fail to gather the information needed to measure progress.

To choose your methodology follow these steps:

- **Select Your Tools** - Choose the assessment tools and measurements that you intend to use to gather data (for example, pain scales, mobility tests, questionnaires).

- **Establish Time Frames** - Decide how often you will track progress—will it be after every session, weekly, or at other intervals? This helps you decide when to collect data and ensures you are capturing meaningful changes.

- **Consistency is Key** - Make sure to use the same methods for tracking progress at every stage of the study to ensure reliability.

Design Your Treatment Plan

Now it is time to create a detailed treatment plan. Your treatment plan is your roadmap for your case study. Without it, you are simply flying blind.

This plan is what you will follow throughout the duration of your case study. It should be based on your client's needs, goals, and the data you have already gathered.

The clearer and more thoughtful your plan, the easier it will be to track progress and achieve your case study goals.

To design your treatment plan, follow these steps:

- **Outline Treatment Techniques** - Based on the assessment, decide which therapeutic techniques you will use. For example, you might choose deep tissue massage, trigger point therapy, stretching, or something else based on the client's condition.

- **Create a Session Schedule** - Consider if you will be doing daily treatments, weekly sessions, or something else? Make sure your treatment plan aligns with the time frames you have set for collecting data and tracking progress.

- **Incorporate Flexibility** - While it is essential to have a plan, it is just as important to remain flexible. You may find that your client's condition evolves in unexpected ways, and your treatment plan should allow for adjustments if needed.

Establish Milestones and Checkpoints

Milestones give you a clear way to measure progress. Without them, it is easy to lose sight of your goals and lose motivation.

You need to break down your case study into smaller milestones to effectively measure progress along the way. These milestones will help you stay on track and evaluate whether your treatment plan is working.

Set milestones as follows:

- **Set Short-Term Milestones** - These could be weekly or bi-weekly targets, such as pain reduction, improved range of motion, or increased energy levels.

- **Long-Term Milestones** - Establish a final goal for the case study, such as achieving a certain percentage of pain relief or a full return to normal function.

- **Regular Progress Assessments** - Schedule periodic evaluations to assess whether you are meeting your milestones. This will allow you to track changes and provide feedback to your client.

Create a Data Collection Framework

Your data collection framework will guide how you gather and organise information over the course of the case study. This is where your baseline measurements, progress assessments, and client feedback will come together.

Having a well-organised framework ensures that you do not miss key details and can easily analyse the data once the case study is complete. A systematic approach to data collection makes it much easier to draw meaningful conclusions at the end of your study.

Create a data collection framework as follows:

- **Decide on the Type of Data** - Are you collecting qualitative data (like client feedback) or quantitative data (like range of motion measurements)? Or both?
- **Create Templates** - Use templates or forms to ensure that you record data is recorded consistently and accurately. For example, you might have a weekly report form for pain levels or progress notes that help you track changes in flexibility.
- **Organise the Data** - Store your data in a way that is easy to analyse later. A spreadsheet like Excel can be a helpful tool for tracking quantitative data, while a client journal can serve as a great repository for qualitative feedback.

For case studies, different types of spreadsheets can help organise data, track progress, and structure findings effectively. Here are some useful spreadsheet types for case study development:

Case Study Planning & Topic Selection Spreadsheet – this helps in brainstorming and evaluating potential case study topics. Columns of this spreadsheet may include Topic ideas, relevance, target journal requirements, expected outcomes, feasibility.

Research & Data Collection Spreadsheet – this organises raw data from observations, client records, or experiments. Columns may include Data source, collection date, variables measured, initial findings.

Patient/Client Information & Progress Tracking Spreadsheet - Records patient/client demographics, symptoms, and treatment progress (for healthcare-related case studies). Columns may include Name/ID, diagnosis, intervention details, progress notes, follow-up status.

Literature Review & References Spreadsheet - Organises relevant research and journal articles for citation. Columns may include Title, author, publication date, key findings, relevance to case study.

Data Analysis & Interpretation Spreadsheet - Used for statistical analysis, trends, and outcome evaluation. Columns may include Pre-treatment vs. post-treatment data, mean values, standard deviation, significance tests.

Ethical Considerations & Compliance Checklist Spreadsheet - Ensures all ethical guidelines and approvals are met. Columns may include Ethical approval status, informed consent obtained, confidentiality measures, conflicts of interest.

Anticipate Potential Challenges

While you can plan every step of your case study, there are always potential challenges that might arise. Whether it is changes in your client's condition or obstacles in tracking data, it is good to be prepared for these.

Anticipating challenges allows you to adjust your design or approach in real time, making your case study more resilient and robust. It also helps you maintain ethical standards and transparency in your work.

Following are some considerations:

- **Consider Client Factors** - Think about your client's commitment to the treatment plan. Are they likely to stick with it, or could external factors (for example, personal commitments or financial constraints) affect the study?

- **Prepare for Data Limitations** - You might run into limitations in how much data you can collect or its accuracy. Be prepared to adapt and make adjustments where necessary. Even if data is not collected at a particular point or about a particular event, it still needs to be documented.

- **Factor in Potential Biases** - Be aware of any biases you might have, either in your treatment approach or in how you interpret the data. Bias can affect the integrity of your case study.

Designing your case study is all about creating a structured plan for both treatment and data collection. By clearly defining your focus, choosing an effective methodology, setting realistic goals and milestones, and preparing for potential challenges, you are setting yourself up for success. A well-designed case study not only helps you achieve meaningful results but also makes it easier to analyse and report those results in a clear, compelling way.

Remember: The more effort you put into designing your case study from the start, the more likely you are to get valuable insights and successful outcomes by the end, and the more likely you are to get it published or accepted for presentation at a conference.

Showing your findings to others may then lead to other more detailed studies or trials.

Build your Blueprint

Think of this step as designing the map before the road trip.

1. **Choose Your Case Study Type:** Are you aiming for an exploratory, descriptive, or explanatory case study? Write down why you chose this approach.
2. **Set Your Timeline:** How long will your case study run? Weeks, months, or longer? Mark some key milestones in your calendar.
3. **Plan Your Documentation Method:** Will you use handwritten notes, digital records, or a client management software?

Does this plan feel doable, or does it need a little fine-tuning?

Page left intentionally blank for your notes.

Conducting the Case Study

Conduct Initial Client Assessment

The first step in creating your case study is the **initial or baseline client assessment**. Think of this step like laying down the first brick of your foundation. A solid assessment gives you all the information you need to create a targeted treatment plan, track progress, and, of course, get results.

The client assessment is about getting to know your client, understanding their goals, and really looking into what is going on with their body. Over the next pages I will highlight what you need to focus on.

Build a Connection

Firstly, get to know your client! Seriously—before you jump into their health history, take a moment to chat. I don't mean a "get through the questions" kind of thing. Building rapport is so important for a successful case study. The more comfortable your client feels with you, the more likely they are to discuss their issues.

Following are some tips for building a connection with your client:

- **Have a Conversation** - Ask open-ended questions like "What's been going on for you lately?" or "What made you decide to get treatment?" It is not just about their condition—it is about understanding who they are and what is going on in their lives.

- **Set the Tone** - Make them feel heard and respected. People are much more likely to share their true concerns if they feel safe and valued.

- **Respect Boundaries** - Be mindful of any personal or sensitive topics. Let them know that they are in control of the conversation.

If your client feels comfortable and valued, they are more likely to be open about their condition. This also sets the stage for you to have a stronger working relationship with your client, which is crucial for a successful outcome.

Gather Client's Health History

After you have established good rapport with your client, it is time to gather their detailed health history. Completing this step gives you the full picture of your client's health. You will want to know about any past injuries, surgeries, and ongoing conditions that could affect their treatment.

Gather the following about the client's health history:

- **Ask About Past Health Issues** - Find out about any surgeries, injuries, or chronic conditions.

This could include everything from a past car accident to conditions like asthma or diabetes.

- **Check for Medications and Allergies** - Be sure to ask about any medications they are taking or known allergies, especially those that might affect your treatments.

- **Lifestyle Factors** - Do not forget to ask about things like their sleep, exercise habits, and stress levels. These can give you some insight into what is going on physically and emotionally.

- **Identify Any Functional Limitations** - Take note of anything that might be affecting their day-to-day life, such as pain, stiffness, or trouble moving.

Understanding your client's health history will help you figure out the best course of action. You want to avoid any treatments that could trigger or worsen existing conditions, and knowing the full scope of their health helps you tailor your approach.

Understand the Main Issue

You can now move on in the process to understand the "heart of the matter": What's the main reason your client is seeking treatment? This is the core of your case study. You want to make sure you fully understand what they are dealing with so you can create a plan to help.

Determine and understand the client's main issue as follows:

- **Let Them Talk About the Issue** - Ask them to describe their symptoms—when did it start, what does it feel like, what makes it better or worse?

- **Pain and Discomfort Levels** - It is helpful to use a pain scale to get a clear picture of how severe the pain is to the client. This gives you a concrete starting point to track changes.

- **Functional Impact** - Find out how the issue is affecting their everyday life. Are they able to do their job? Can they exercise? Knowing the real-life impact will guide your treatment choices.

Understanding the specific issue gives you the focus you need to move forward. The clearer the problem is, the better you can measure progress and success as you work through the case study.

Set SMART Goals

This is where you and your client can really start collaborating. What are they hoping to get out of treatment? It is not enough to just say, "I want to feel better." You need clear, actionable goals—goals that are **SMART** (Specific, Measurable, Achievable, Relevant, and Time-bound).

Set the SMART goals as follows:

- **Discuss Their Desired Outcome** - What do they want to achieve? It could be reducing pain, improving mobility, or simply feeling more energetic. Get clarity on this.

- **Set SMART Goals** - For example, instead of "reduce pain," you might set a goal like, "Reduce pain from a 7/10 to a 4/10 in the next 3 weeks."

- **Break It Down** - Big goals can feel overwhelming. Break them down into smaller, achievable milestones. That way, you and your client can celebrate small wins along the way.

Setting clear goals helps both you and your client know what success looks like. It gives you something to measure against, and it helps keep your treatment focused and on track.

Conduct Physical and Functional Assessments

At this point you will need to be more hands-on. You should start collecting the physical data that will serve as your baseline. From range of motion to posture, these assessments help you understand where things are right now—and how much they improve over time.

Complete these physical and functional assessments:

- **Check Range of Motion** – Determine how flexible or stiff the client is in certain joints and areas of their body. This helps you pinpoint where they might be limited.

- **Assess Strength** - You can assess muscle strength or imbalances that might be affecting the client's condition.
- **Posture Check** - Notice any postural issues that could be contributing to the problem, like rounded shoulders or misaligned hips.

- **Functional Movement Screen** - If relevant, use a functional movement screen to see how your client moves and identify any specific patterns causing pain.

These assessments give you solid data on where your client's starting point. Having this baseline allows you to track progress and adjust your treatment plan as needed.

Create a Client Profile

Once you have gathered all the details, it is time to pull everything together into a **client profile**. This will be your go-to reference throughout the case study, helping you stay organised and focused.

Create a client profile as follows:

- **Summarise Their Health History** - Put together a quick summary of relevant health conditions, past injuries, and lifestyle factors.

- **Highlight the Primary Issue** - Make sure the main complaint is clear, along with any functional limitations they are experiencing.

- **List Their SMART Goals** - Write down the goals you have agreed on with your client.

- **Include Assessment Findings** - Document all the physical assessments you have done, so you have a clear starting point for tracking progress.

Having a well-organised profile helps you stay on track throughout the case study. It is also a helpful reference when you need to adjust your treatment plan or when you are reporting on the outcomes.

The goal of the initial client assessment is to obtain a clear, comprehensive picture of your client's health and their goals. With this solid foundation, you will be in a much better position to create a targeted, effective treatment plan. And as you move through the case study, you will have this information to guide your decisions and measure success.

Remember: the more thorough and thoughtful your initial assessment, the better your case study will be. It also sets you up for success as you collaborate with your client to achieve their goals. Take your time to ask the right questions, and most importantly, listen to what your client is telling you. They are the key to unlocking a successful treatment plan.

Exercise

1. **Perform the Assessment:** Use your checklist from this chapter and gather baseline data. Observe posture, range of motion, areas of tension, and client-reported symptoms.
2. **Record Your Findings:** Write detailed notes – remember, clarity now saves headaches later.
3. **Take Baseline Photos (if applicable):** Take initial photographs (with detailed written consent) to capture visual data.

What was the most surprising or revealing thing you learned during this assessment?

Page left intentionally blank for your notes.

Implementing Treatment Plans

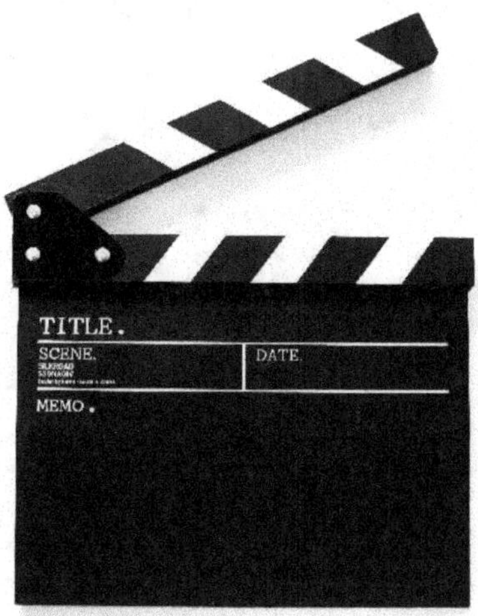

After gathering all the information from your initial assessment, it is time to put that knowledge into action with your **treatment plan**. *Think of this as your game plan—it is what will guide your treatments, track your client's progress, and ultimately help them achieve their goals.*

But creating a treatment plan is not a one-size-fits-all process. You must tailor it to your client's unique needs, their goals, and what you have learned from the assessment. It is like making a personalised roadmap—if you do not know where you are going, how can you get there?

Review the Gathered Information

Before you start drafting your plan, take a moment to revisit all the details from the initial assessment. Remember, you have built the treatment plan based on the foundation of your client's history, their goals, and the initial assessments that you conducted. Take time and do not rush through building your treatment plan to ensure you thoroughly cover your client's issues.

Revisit the **client profile** you created in the initial assessment. Review the information to ensure you have a clear understanding of the client's primary concerns and their SMART goals.

Reflect on the physical and functional assessments you completed. Are there any patterns or red flags that you need to be mindful of?

The more you understand your client's starting point, the more accurately you can design a treatment plan that addresses their needs. You want this plan to be laser-focused on their individual goals, not just a generic treatment template.

Set Realistic and Achievable Goals

During the assessment phase you will have applied SMART goals. Now it is time to refine and set actionable treatment goals that fit the bigger picture.

These goals should not only be **specific** and **measurable**, but also **achievable** and **time bound**. Keep in mind the resources and time you have available to work with!

You need to consider the following: format

- **Break Down the Big Goals** – If your client's goal is "to reduce pain," break that down into smaller, measurable goals like "reduce pain from a 7/10 to a 4/10 in three weeks."

- **Consider Timeframes** - How long do you have to work with the client? It is crucial that the goals are achievable within your timeframe.

- **Stay Flexible** - Things may change along the way, so make sure your goals allow for flexibility. Life happens!

Setting clear, realistic goals gives you direction, and it gives your client something to look forward to. It also allows you to celebrate the small wins along the way, which keeps motivation high.

Choose Appropriate Treatment Techniques

Based on your client's condition, health history, and goals, you will need to determine the treatment options that will be effective and appropriate to your client. This where your expertise really comes into play.

Following outlines the method:

- **Tailor Your Approach:** The techniques you choose should align with your client's primary issue. For example, if their main concern is muscle stiffness, you might incorporate deep tissue massage or myofascial release. If stress is a factor, relaxation techniques like aromatherapy or Swedish massage could be a better fit.
- **Consider any Contraindications.** Be sure you are aware of any contraindications or precautions based on the client's health history. If they have had a recent surgery, for instance, you would not want to use techniques that put too much pressure on the area.

Your treatment techniques need to be both effective and safe. Selecting the right combination of techniques will help you to achieve the best possible outcomes.

Design a Treatment Schedule

Once you have figured out what techniques you are going to use, you need to map out the **treatment**

schedule. How many sessions do you need? How often should they be scheduled? And how long should each session last? This schedule will depend on the client's condition and goals, as well as their availability.

Frequency and Duration

For an acute issue, you might need to see your client more frequently (2-3 times a week). For chronic conditions, once a week or bi-weekly might suffice.

Progress Checkpoints

Set specific times in the schedule to check in on the client's progress. This gives both you and your client a chance to assess how things are going and adjust if needed.

Having a clear schedule keeps you on track. Plus, regular check-ins help you gauge progress and tweak your treatment as needed.

Incorporate Client Feedback

As you start collaborating with your client, do not forget to check in with them regularly. The treatment plan is not a rigid, unchanging blueprint—it is a living document that should adapt based on your client's feedback.

Ask questions after every session. Find out what worked, what did not, and how they are feeling. Ask them if anything caused discomfort or if they noticed any improvements.

Make Adjustments*. If something is not working, you can change your approach. Sometimes a certain technique is too intense. Client feedback is key.

Client feedback is invaluable in shaping the course of treatment. It ensures you are meeting the client's needs and adjusting treatment when necessary. It also helps build trust because your client sees that you are actively working with them to achieve the best outcomes.

* Keep in mind when "Making Adjustments" not to change measurement parameters to suit a biased hypothesis, thus bringing the study's integrity into question.

Document Everything

Throughout the process, make sure you are keeping detailed notes on everything. You should document every treatment session, every adjustment, and every piece of feedback. This will not only help you track progress, but it will also be useful for any follow-up care or future case studies.

Following are some tips:

- **Record Treatment Details** - Write down what you did during each session, including any techniques used, areas treated, and how the client responded.

- **Track Progress** - Use your initial assessments and goals as benchmarks to document changes over time.

- **Note Adjustments** - If you tweak the treatment plan based on client feedback, make sure that you record this as well.

Documenting everything allows you to reflect on the journey and ensure that you are staying on track. It also provides a valuable record for future reference or case studies.

Let the participant(s) know what you are documenting and ask perhaps if there is other information that they think would be worth collecting about them or the intervention.

Evaluate and Adjust as You Go

The treatment plan should not be static—it needs to evolve based on how your client responds. Regular evaluations will help you determine if the plan is working or if you need to make any changes.

Review Progress Periodically

Set milestones (for example, after three weeks, six weeks, etc.) to check on progress. Are they feeling better? Is the treatment meeting the client's goals?

Adjust as Needed

If something is not working, change it. Record any changes and the reason for them and always assess for bias. Whether it is adjusting the techniques, changing the treatment schedule, or reassessing the goals, be flexible!

Evaluating and adjusting keeps your treatment plan aligned with the client's needs and helps you reach the goal: a successful outcome.

To implement an effective treatment plan it is all about taking the information you gathered from the initial assessment and turning it into a targeted, flexible approach that meets the client's needs. You will need to continually adapt and refine your plan based on their feedback and progress, and by the end of the case study, you will have a solid record of everything you have done.

Remember, your treatment plan is your blueprint—but it is not set in stone. You must be flexible and modify and tailor it with your client's changing needs and feedback in order for it to be successful.

Time to Put the Treatment Plan in Motion

This is where the magic happens.

- **Write Down Your Plan -** Outline your treatment goals, the techniques you will use, and your expected outcomes.

- **Start the First Session -** Document what you did, how the client responded, and any initial observations.

- **Adjust if Needed -** After the session, reflect on whether your plan feels solid or needs tweaks.

How did your client respond to the first session, and did it match your expectations?

Page left intentionally blank for your notes.

Monitoring Progress

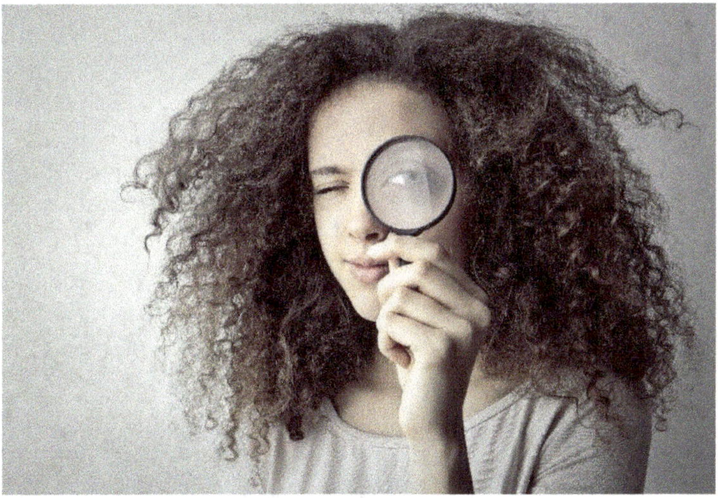

Photo by Olly

Monitoring progress is one of the most crucial steps in a case study because it helps you stay on track, ensures your treatment plan is working, and gives you insights into how you can adjust your approach if needed. Think of it as your regular check-in to see if things are moving in the right direction. It is not just about tracking numbers—it is about understanding the ***journey*** *your client is on and how you can help them move forward.*

Keep an Eye on Change

Monitoring progress is one of the most critical aspects of conducting a successful case study – without it you are flying blind. By recording and tracking the progress you can see whether your treatment plan is effective by observing patterns; identify areas that may need modification and make informed adjustments as your progress; and ensure that your approach aligns with your client's evolving needs.

When we monitor progress consistently, we gather valuable data that tells a story over time. Instead of relying on memory or subjective impressions, you will have objective evidence to demonstrate changes—whether they are improvements, plateaus, or unexpected outcomes. This documentation can also reveal trends that might not have been obvious in a single session, helping you refine your techniques or adapt your plan for better results.

Additionally, tracking progress builds trust and transparency with your clients. When you can show measurable improvements or explain why adjustments are being made, it reassures clients that their well-being is at the center of your care. For example, noting changes in scar tissue mobility, range of motion, or pain levels over time allows both you and your client to see tangible results, which can be incredibly motivating and empowering.

From a research perspective, detailed progress monitoring strengthens the credibility of your findings. It provides a clear timeline of interventions, responses, and outcomes, ensuring your case study isn't just anecdotal but grounded in evidence. Whether you are using assessment tools, photographic records, or client feedback forms, every piece of data contributes to the bigger picture.

In short, monitoring progress is the bridge between intention and outcome. It is how we validate our work, refine our methods, and ensure our case studies offer meaningful insights to the wider massage therapy community.

To summarise, monitoring progress helps you assess the effectiveness of your treatment. Are your chosen techniques working as expected?

It helps you track changes over time. Is your client improving, staying the same, or experiencing setbacks?

Monitoring progress also helps you adjust the plan. If something is not working, you can tweak your approach to get better results.

So, it is not just about the initial results—it is about **continuous improvement** and making sure you are providing the best care possible.

Set Up Progress Indicators

Before beginning treatment, you must determine how you will measure progress. These indicators will help you evaluate whether the client is heading toward their goals. They can be **quantitative** (like pain levels, range of motion, or muscle strength) or **qualitative** (like the client's perception of how they are feeling or how their symptoms impact their daily life). Both are valuable, so don't underestimate the value of either.

Choose Specific Metrics

As an example, if your client is experiencing pain, you could use a pain scale (0-10) to track changes. If their goal is to increase flexibility, a simple test of range of motion might work.

Even in a case study, it is crucial to use validated tools or instruments to ensure the accuracy, reliability, and credibility of the data collected. Using well-established measurement methods enhances the study's scientific rigor, allows for meaningful comparisons with existing research, and increases the likelihood of publication in reputable journals. Without validated tools, findings may be questioned or considered anecdotal rather than evidence based.

Include Client Feedback

While numbers are useful, do not forget to consider how the client feels about their progress. Maybe your client feels more relaxed, is less stressed, or has noticed fewer headaches.

Having a clear set of indicators will give you a concrete way to measure progress and will help you stay focused on the client's goals.

Track Progress Over Time

Consistency is vital in tracking progress. You need to keep detailed records of each session and document any changes in the client's condition or symptoms. This helps you identify trends over time. Is the client steadily improving? Are there any plateaus or setbacks?

After each session, jot down observations. Did the client report any pain or discomfort? Were there any changes in their mobility or posture? What treatments did you use, and how did they respond?

You can also use charts or logs to visually track changes over time. Seeing that steady improvement on paper can be a real motivator for both you and your client.

Tracking this information helps you stay organised and gives you a clear overview of how things are progressing. It is like having a road map to follow, helping you adjust treatment when needed.

Check-in with the Client Regularly

Progress is not just about what you observe during the treatment sessions—it is also about **how the client feels** in between sessions. Regular check-ins help you gauge whether the treatment is truly working from the client's perspective. It also builds trust because the client feels heard and understood.

Ask open-ended questions. Don't just ask, "How do you feel?" Ask more specific questions like, "Have you noticed any changes in your pain levels since our last session?" or "Have you been able to perform any activities that were previously difficult?"

Encourage open communication. Let your client know that they should feel comfortable sharing their thoughts and concerns at any point in the process. This creates a supportive environment where you are both invested in the success of the treatment.

The client's perspective can give you valuable insights that you might not notice during treatment. Plus, it fosters a sense of collaboration, which is key for getting the best results.

Adjust the Treatment Plan

As you monitor progress, be prepared to adjust your treatment plan as needed. Sometimes, the original plan works as desired; other times, you may need to tweak things based on what you are seeing and hearing from your client.

Evaluate the plan regularly. After a set number of sessions with your client (for example, every 3-4 weeks), review the progress you have made toward the goals. Are they on track? Is something not working?

Make adjustments to the treatment plan if needed. You can adjust the treatment techniques, session frequency, or even the goals themselves, based on client feedback, progress tracking, or new observations.

Your goal should be to ensure treatment plan stays effective and relevant to your client's needs. No two clients are the same, and being flexible shows that you are dedicated to their journey.

Record outcomes (whether they support your hypothesis or not). Assess any adjustments for bias. Record adjustments. Implement adjustments. Maintain the integrity of all of your hard work!

Reassess and Reconfirm the Goals

Sometimes, as the case study progresses, you might find that the initial goals are no longer aligned with what the client needs. This is not a bad thing—it is just a natural part of the process.

Revisit the SMART Goals

After a few sessions, sit down with your client and review their goals. Are they still relevant? Do they need to be adjusted based on the progress made so far?

Refine as Needed

If the original goals have been met, celebrate that success and set new goals! Or, if progress has been slower than expected, you may want to modify the goals to make them more realistic.

Reassessing the goals keeps both you and your client focused and aligned. It ensures you are always working toward what matters most to your client, and it helps maintain motivation as you continue to see progress.

Reflect on Progress

Finally, take some time to reflect on the progress made throughout the case study. This reflection process is not just about your client—it is also about you. You will want to evaluate how you have handled the case, what you have learned, and what you can improve in future cases.

After completing the case study, review your treatment plan and your progress notes. What worked well? What could you have done differently?

It is important to celebrate your client's progress (no matter how big or small) as well as your own growth as a practitioner. This is a learning journey for both of you.

Reflection is essential for growth. Not only does it help you improve as a therapist, but it also deepens your understanding of how to tailor treatment plans and monitor progress effectively.

When you monitor progress, you are keeping a close eye on the client's journey and adjusting their treatment plan as needed. It is like having a built-in feedback loop that ensures you are always working toward the best possible outcomes. By tracking specific indicators, checking in with the client regularly, and being flexible in your approach, you can ensure that your case study remains on track and focused on achieving the client's goals. Remember to celebrate the little victories along the way.

Keep an Eye on the Journey

Progress tracking does not have to be complicated – it just needs to be consistent. Remember these factors:

- **Choose Your Metrics -** Are you tracking pain levels, mobility, mood, or something else? Write them down.

- **Set a Routine -** Decide how often you will check in on these metrics – every session, every week?

- **Document Diligently** - Create a simple log where you can jot down observations after each session.

What small wins have you noticed so far, and how do they encourage you? What did not go to plan and was a disappointment? Where there any unexpected outcomes?

Page left intentionally blank for your notes.

Documenting The Process

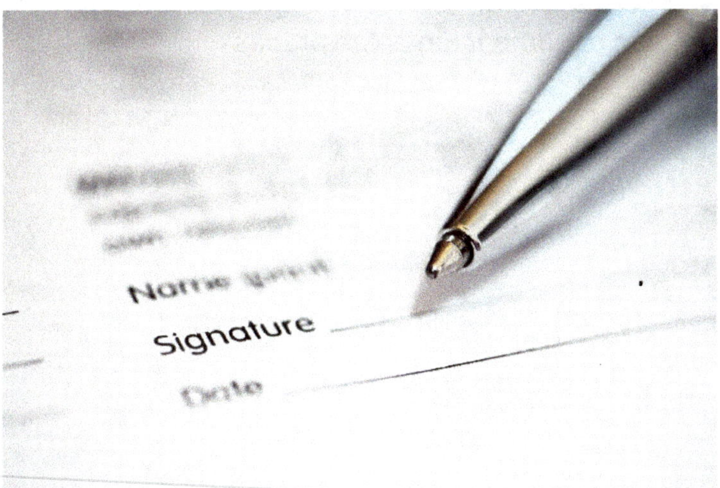

Documenting the process of your case study is like keeping a diary of everything that happens throughout the journey. It is more than just jotting down facts—it is about capturing the story of your client's progress, the treatment choices you made, and the results that followed. In a nutshell, approach it as a way of providing a thorough, transparent account of the case from start to finish.

Documenting does not have to be a chore. It is the most important method for reflecting on the process and proving that the treatment you provided had real, measurable results. So, let's see why and how you should document the entire process.

Why is documentation so important

Think of your case study as a blueprint for your future practice. Documentation is not just about checking a box; it serves several critical purposes.

It keeps you organised. When you document every step of the process, you are building a roadmap. It helps you keep track of what has been done, what is working, and where adjustments are needed.

Good documentation supports your conclusions. The more you document, the stronger your case study will be. Good documentation shows the reasoning behind your treatment choices and the results, making your conclusions much more credible.

It also helps with accountability. You are not just working with your client's health—you are also working with your own professional reputation. By documenting everything, you protect yourself and your practice by showing you are following through on your treatment plans and goals.

By recording your thoughts and observations throughout the case, you create a resource you can refer to. It is a great way to reflect on what went well, what could be improved, and how you can apply the lessons learned to future cases.

What to Document

This section outlines what information you should be documenting in the case study. When documenting a case study, choose a method that best suits your workflow—whether typing your notes, using voice-to-text software, or recording audio or video reflections. Typing ensures clarity and easy organisation, while speaking your observations into a voice recorder or transcription app can capture real-time insights without interrupting the flow of work. If using recordings, be sure to transcribe key details and securely store the files to maintain accuracy and confidentiality.

Client Information

To build the foundation of your case study you will need to record important client details such as:

- **Personal information** - Name, age, occupation, contact information, etc.
- **Medical history** - include any previous diagnoses, treatments, and surgeries related to their condition.
- **Current complaints** - What brought them to your practice? Be as detailed as possible here—include specifics on pain, mobility issues, or other symptoms.

Initial Assessment and Findings

Establish your baseline during the initial assessment, and document:

- **Posture and movement analysis** - Describe how the client's posture looks and any noticeable dysfunctions or limitations in movement.

- **Symptom analysis** - Document any pain or discomfort the client is experiencing and where it is located, along with the severity.

- **Treatment goals** - Outline what the client hopes to achieve through treatment. These should be clear and measurable (using the SMART framework we discussed earlier).

Treatment Plan

Develop a treatment plan which records the steps you are going to take to address the client's needs:

- **Techniques and modalities used**
  Describe the treatments and techniques you plan to use. Whether it is a specific massage technique or a set of stretches, this is where you detail the approach.

- **Frequency and duration of treatment**

Note how often you will be seeing the client and for how long each session will last.

- **Expected outcomes**
  What are the anticipated results based on your treatment plan? These should tie back to the client's goals.

Session Notes

For each session, you should record the following:

- **What was done during the session** - Include the techniques used, any observations, and any changes to the treatment plan.

- **Client's feedback** - Document how the client felt before, during, and after the session. Did they report less pain, more movement, or a different symptom.

- **Any changes or adjustment** - If the client's condition has changed since the last session (for better or worse), note that down. You may need to adjust the treatment plan accordingly.

- **Before and After Photos** - We will cover this in more detail in the next chapter.

Progress and Adjustments

As the case study progresses, document how things evolve:

- **Progress toward goals** - Track improvements or setbacks. Did the client's pain levels decrease? Are they able to move more freely? How does this compare to the initial assessment?

- **Modifications to the treatment plan** - If the client's condition changes or new challenges arise, be sure to document how you modify the treatment plan in response.

How to Document Effectively

You do not need to write a novel for every session, but keeping clear, concise, and consistent records will go a long way. Here are a few tips to make the process easier:

Be Consistent

The key to effective documentation is consistency. Whether you are writing by hand or using an electronic health record (EHR) system, you need to stick to the same format every time. This will help you stay organised and ensure nothing important slips through the cracks.

Utilise a standard template for your notes. This can be a physical form or a digital template in your EHR system.

Make sure you create specific sections for each aspect of the case (for example, assessment, treatment, progress, feedback.

Be Objective and Accurate

In your documentation you need to aim for clarity and precision. Avoid vague or overly subjective terms like “feels better” or “seems fine.” Instead, use measurable terms (like pain scale ratings, range of motion, etc.) that are objective and easy to track.

You should stick to facts—what you saw, heard, and observed.

Also use numbers when possible (for example, pain levels from 1 to 10, range of motion in degrees).

Protect Client Privacy

Confidentiality is crucial when documenting client information. Whether you are storing notes on paper or digitally, ensure that you are following appropriate privacy guidelines to keep your client’s data safe.

Keep all records in a secure location, whether that is a locked file cabinet for physical documents or password-protected files for digital records.

You need to be mindful of the information you are sharing. Avoid including personal details in notes that are not relevant to the treatment.

Review Your Documentation

After you have written up the details, take some time to review everything before moving on to the next phase of the case study. Double-check that all the essential information is there and that your documentation aligns with the treatment goals.

- **Check for completeness** - Did you cover all aspects of the case, from initial assessment to treatment plan and progress?

- **Look for patterns** - As you review, you might spot emerging patterns that help guide your future treatment decisions.

- **Be honest about setbacks** - If something did not go as planned, document it. It is important to capture the full picture—not just the successes.

Documenting your case study might seem like a time-consuming task at first, but trust me, it is worth it. Not only does it help you stay organised and ensure that you are meeting your client's needs, but it also provides a roadmap for you to refer back to in future cases. Plus, good documentation supports your professional credibility by showing that you are following a well-thought-out, methodical process.

When you document your case study thoroughly, you are doing more than just recording what is happening—you are creating a valuable resource that helps both you and your client get the best possible results.

Details, Details, Details

Good documentation is like a trail of breadcrumbs – it makes your study easier to follow.

1. **Create a Template:** Design a standard format for your session notes. Include date, techniques used, observations, and client feedback.

2. **Be Consistent:** Use this format for your next session and see how it feels.

3. **Organise Your Notes:** Decide where and how you will store these records securely.

If someone else read your notes, would they understand your process clearly?

Page left intentionally blank for your notes.

Photography and Video

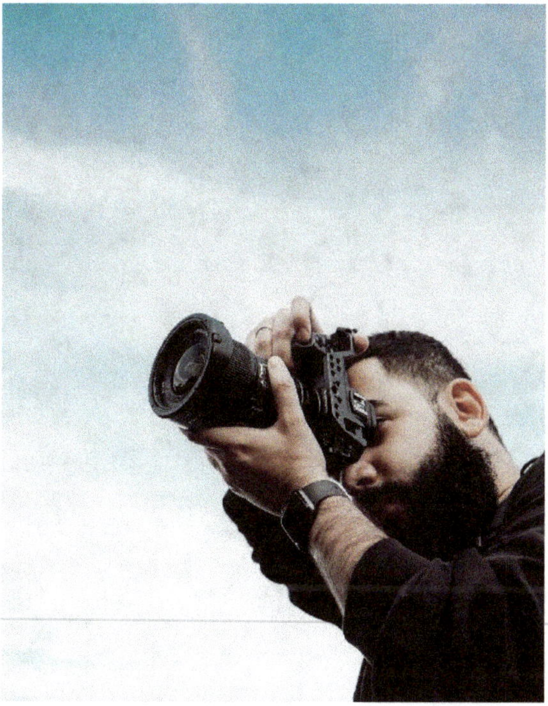

Photo by Aidiramdphoto

Photography *can really enhance the depth of your documentation in so far as they can be a game-changer. They capture the details that words cannot always convey and provide a visual reference that helps you, your client, and anyone reviewing the case study to see progress and changes more clearly.*

This section discusses the importance of photography in documenting and analysing your case study as well as the ethical and practical considerations involved.

Using Images in Documentation

Photos are powerful. They can tell a story, highlight key moments, and give you a snapshot (literally) of your client's condition at various points in the case. This section outlines why it is so beneficial to include photos in your case study.

Visual Evidence of Change

Sometimes, it is hard for both you and your client to really see improvement in real-time. When you compare photos taken at various stages of treatment, it becomes clear how far your client has improved. This is especially helpful with conditions like postural issues, swelling, or muscle tone changes, where visual progress can be more dramatic than the changes that the clients feel.

For example, if you are working with a client who has a chronic pain issue, taking photos of their posture, affected areas, or visible symptoms at the start of treatment and then again after several sessions can show a tangible improvement. This not only boosts your client's confidence but also helps you assess your treatment effectiveness.

Clarifies Observations

Sometimes words just do not do justice to a condition. A photo can highlight areas of tension, swelling, bruising, or joint deformities that may not be immediately obvious from a description. It helps to paint a clearer picture for anyone reviewing your case study—whether that is a colleague, a supervisor, or a student learning from your work.

Let's say a client has a visible injury. A photo can document the severity of the injury or the condition over time, which can be invaluable when discussing treatment options or outcomes with others.

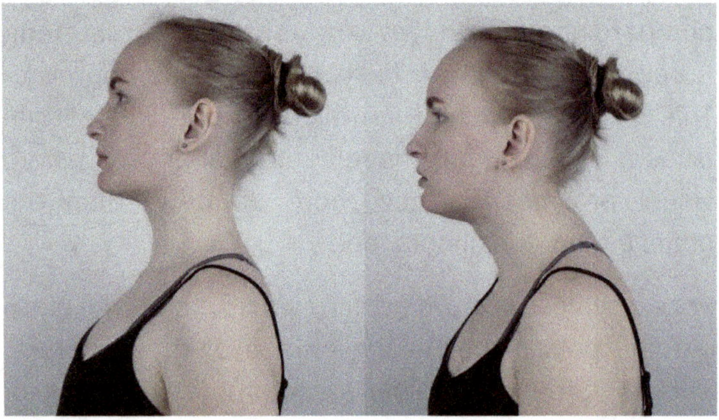

In this photo example the change of posture is clearly visible. The right photo was taken before treatment, and the left photo shows improvement in posture after treatment.

Supports Documentation and Reflection

Including photos as part of your documentation process can make your notes more comprehensive and relatable. You do not have to describe every detail when you have a visual reference that speaks for itself. Looking back at photos helps you reflect on your treatment decisions and the effectiveness of your methods.

For instance, if a client's mobility improves after a series of treatments, reviewing photos showing their range of motion at different points can help you evaluate whether your treatment plan was successful or whether adjustments are needed.

Best Practices for Using Photography

This section discusses how to take and use photos effectively. One thing to remember is that you do not need to be a professional photographer. You can you use mobile phone camera to take some reasonable pictures.

Get Client Consent

It is vital to obtain your client's consent. Always ask for your client's permission before taking any photos. Explain how the photos will be used—whether they will be part of your case study, for documentation purposes, or for teaching others. Your client has a right to privacy, and respecting that consent is crucial.

Have your client sign a consent form.

Be transparent about how and where the photos will be used, ensuring confidentiality if the photos will be shared publicly or used for educational purposes.

Use a Consistent Method

For your photos to be useful in the case study, they need to be taken consistently. Make sure you are using the same angles, lighting, and framing every time you capture an image. This will help you track progress more effectively and ensure the photos serve as reliable references.

Take photos from the same angle every time (for example, front, side, or back view) to maintain consistency. It may be useful to take photos at some distance as well so later they can be superimposed onto others to see any change.

Use a neutral background that does not distract from the subject.

Ensure good lighting so that the photos are clear, and the details are visible.

Show the Full Picture

Make sure that the photos accurately represent what you are treating. If you are documenting an injury, pain area, or posture, take photos that show the entire relevant area so you can track changes over time. If you are focusing on a specific issue, like swelling in the legs, make sure the photo captures the affected area in full view.

If you are documenting a client's posture, take full-body photos (front and side) that show the entire body in relation to the ground.

For injuries or swelling, make sure to capture the whole area, not just the symptomatic spots.

Document Date and Time

It is essential to document when each photo was taken so you can accurately track the progress or changes over time. You can do this by adding a timestamp or simply noting the date and session number to the photo in your case study documentation. This will can help contextualise the photos and match them with your treatment notes.

Keep a record of each session, so you can match each image with the treatment and progress during that time.

Be Mindful of Sensitivity

Some clients may not be comfortable with having their photos taken, especially if the condition being treated is sensitive or personal. Always approach this with respect and ensure your client feels comfortable and in control of the process. If a client is not comfortable with photographs, there are alternative ways to document their progress.

Alternative approaches you can offer your client if they are uncomfortable with photos include detailed notes or sketches of the areas being treated.

Respect your client's wishes and provide reassurance if needed.

Ethical Considerations in Photography

While photography can be incredibly valuable, it also comes with ethical considerations, especially when it comes to client privacy, consent, and the potential for misuse. This section covers some of the key ethical principles.

Confidentiality

Make sure that any photos you take are kept secure and used appropriately. If your case study will be shared or published, you may need to anonymise photos or blur out identifiable features to protect your client's identity.

Store photos securely, whether on a private server, encrypted cloud storage, or locked file storage.

If you are using the photos for teaching or publication, ensure that any identifying information is removed to protect your client's confidentiality.

Informed Consent

This cannot be emphasised enough. Always get written permission before photographing your client, especially if you plan to use the images for educational purposes, publication, or in any manner that goes beyond the initial case study documentation.

For more information on Consent forms refer to the section on consent.

Use Photos for Professional Purposes Only

Do not use photos of your clients for personal gain or in ways that could make them feel uncomfortable.

Only use photos in professional, educational, or case-study contexts where your client has agreed.

Avoid sharing or posting images on social media unless you have obtained full consent from your client.

Incorporating photography into your case study can elevate your documentation and offer a visual testament to the changes and progress your client makes. But like any powerful tool, it should be used thoughtfully and ethically. By following best practices and respecting client privacy, you can ensure that photography becomes an asset to your case study process—helping you document, reflect, and communicate more effectively.

With the right approach, photography can be a fantastic way to bring your case study to life—capturing every moment of the journey.

A Picture's Worth a Thousand Words

1. **Take Follow-Up Photos:** Capture progress points (with client consent). Think posture, swelling, or other visible changes.
2. **Label and Store Photos:** Make sure each image is dated and connected to session notes.
3. **Reflect on Visuals:** What do these images tell you about your client's journey?

How do these photos enhance your written documentation?

Page left intentionally blank for your notes.

Referencing in Case Studies

Pluck, A. (2024). Improvement in quality of life and speech: Case study of a head and neck cancer patient using manual lymphatic drainage and bioelectric massage therapy. *Journal of Lymphoedema*, *19*(1).

When you are conducting a case study, it is essential to back up your observations, treatments, and conclusions with credible sources. This is where referencing comes into play. Not only does referencing add credibility to your work, but it also helps you demonstrate that your decisions are grounded in proven techniques, established research, or expert opinions.

But referencing does not have to feel like a chore. Think of it as a way of crediting the hard work of others and show your audience that you're building on a solid foundation of knowledge. This section outlines why referencing is so important, how to do it effectively, and where it fits into your case study.

The Importance of Referencing

As a professional massage therapist, you have a wealth of knowledge and experience. But when you are documenting your case study, referencing external sources reinforces your integrity and professionalism. It shows that your treatment plans and approaches are not just based on anecdotal evidence but are supported by credible evidence and industry best practices.

For example, when you reference a study that supports a particular massage technique or the efficacy of a certain modality, you are demonstrating that your choices are not arbitrary. This can inspire confidence in anyone who reads your case study.

Referencing helps build credibility and trust.

Validates Your Findings

In a case study, you are documenting your own and your client's journey. It is vital that the observations and conclusions you draw are not only personal but also reflective of broader knowledge and established findings in the field. References provide the scientific backing or expert opinions that lend weight to your treatment plans, observations, and conclusions.

Imagine you have identified a noticeable improvement in your client's flexibility after using a particular technique. By referencing studies or articles that show this same technique's effectiveness, you provide solid support for your conclusion, making your findings more convincing.

Provides a Learning Resource

A good case study does not just end with the results; it should also educate the reader. When you reference studies, articles, or textbooks, you are offering a pathway for others to explore the topic more deeply. For example, if you are discussing a specialised treatment method, referencing the source allows your reader to learn more about it if they are interested. This turns your case study into a resource.

How to Reference Effectively

The references you choose should be directly relevant to the case study you are writing. Do not feel the need to fill your references list with every book or article you have ever read. Stick to the key sources that directly support your findings, methods, or conclusions.

Always choose relevant and credible sources.

Refer to peer-reviewed journals, textbooks from experts in the field, and credible websites (like professional associations or educational platforms).

If referencing a case study, be sure it is relevant and supports the points you are making about your own practice.

Be Consistent with Your Referencing Style

Consistency is key when it comes to referencing. Different publications and institutions prefer different referencing styles, but the key is to stick to one style throughout your case study. Whether you are using APA (American Psychological Association), MLA (Modern Language Association), or any other style, make sure you follow the rules closely for citing sources, especially when it comes to formatting, in-text citations, and your reference list.

Decide on a referencing style before you start writing and stick with it throughout the report. Of course, referencing style may also be dependent on the journal you have decided to publish in.

Include complete details for each reference—author names, publication years, titles, and source information.

Incorporate References into Your Writing Smoothly

When referencing in your case study, do not just throw in citations where you think they fit. Seamlessly integrate them into your writing so they support your narrative without interrupting the flow. This keeps your case study engaging while reinforcing the evidence behind your decisions.

For example, instead of just saying, "I used myofascial release," you could say, "Myofascial release, as supported by Smith (2020), was chosen for its ability to target chronic muscle tension in the upper back." This way, you are not only explaining your choice but showing that it is based on evidence.

Balance Between Personal Experience and External Sources

Remember, the case study is about your experience collaborating with your client. You do not want to lose your personal touch by overloading the study with references. However, blending your own observations with credible research is a powerful way to show both practical application and scholarly rigor.

Share your observations and conclusions but reinforce them with references that back up your decisions and treatment plans.

Do not be afraid to cite your own evidence based, peer-reviewed work, especially if you have published studies or articles on the subject.

Where to Include References

In your case study, you can use references in the following ways:

Background and Theory Section

This is where you set the stage and explain the concepts and theories behind your treatment methods. References in this section could include research articles or textbooks that explain the techniques or approaches you will be using.

For example:

- "Massage therapy, especially deep tissue techniques, has been shown to help alleviate chronic pain in the neck and shoulders (Jones et al., 2021)."

Treatment Plan Section

When you explain why you have chosen a particular treatment for your client, this is the perfect place to include references to studies or articles that support the effectiveness of that treatment.

For example:

- "The use of heat therapy, as recommended by Smith (2022), can enhance muscle relaxation and reduce inflammation, making it a suitable addition to the treatment plan."

Analysis and Outcome Section

In this part of the case study, you will discuss the progress of your client and how the treatment is working. Here, you can refer to research that shows how the techniques you have used typically result in certain outcomes, whether that is increased flexibility, reduced pain, or other improvements.

For example:

- "Following a regimen of manual lymphatic drainage, as outlined by the Australasian Lymphology Association (2019), clients typically report significant reduction in swelling within two weeks of treatment."

Conclusion and Reflection

At the end of your case study, you will likely reflect on the overall process, what worked well, and what could be improved. This is a suitable time to include references that highlight trends or observations you have made based on evidence in the field.

For example:

- "While the client showed significant improvement, further studies on the long-term effects of combined treatments (Green et al., 2020) suggest that incorporating regular follow-ups may help sustain these benefits."

Common Pitfalls to Avoid in Referencing

You need to ensure that you don't overcite but also you should cite your own published works.

Over-Citing

It can be tempting to reference every piece of material you have read on the topic, but too many references can overwhelm your case study and distract from your primary message. Keep it focused on what directly supports your work.

Focus on making sure that every reference you include genuinely enhances your study.

Not Citing Your Own Work

If you have published studies or have firsthand experience that contributes to the case study, do not be afraid to reference your own work. This not only shows confidence in your experience but also reinforces your integrity and professionalism.

Incorporating references into your case study is not just about making it look more scholarly—it is about providing the foundation and credibility your treatment decisions are based on. The references you choose should back up your findings and conclusions, giving your case study depth and context.

When done right, referencing is a powerful tool that elevates your work from anecdotal to evidence-based, showing your commitment to providing the best possible care for your clients.

So, next time you are writing a case study, remember that referencing is not a task—it is an opportunity to demonstrate the knowledge that underpins your practice and ensure your work stands the test of time.

Time to Show Your Sources

Citations are not just for academics – they build credibility.

1. **Gather References:** Find 2–3 credible sources related to your topic (for example, research articles, textbooks).
2. **Create a Reference List:** Write them out in the correct format (APA, MLA, or your preferred style).
3. **Integrate into Your Work:** Identify where these references might support your findings.

How do these references add weight to your study?

Page left intentionally blank for your notes.

Analysing and Reporting Findings

Data Analysis Techniques

Once you have gathered the data from your case study, the next step is analysing it. This is where the magic happens—turning raw information into insights that help you understand the effects of your treatments and draw meaningful conclusions. The data analysis techniques you choose will depend on the type of data you have collected (quantitative or qualitative), the objectives of your case study, and the level of detail you need to uncover patterns or trends.

There are different data analysis techniques you can use, and I will guide you through how to approach them in a practical, no-fuss way.

Quantitative Data Analysis

Quantitative data is all about numbers—think measurements, scales, and any data you can measure or quantify. For example, you might have collected data on your client's pain levels, range of motion, or swelling reduction over time. To analyse this data, you will often use statistical methods to identify trends, differences, or correlations.

Key Techniques for Quantitative Data

Descriptive Statistics

These are the basics—the numbers that summarise your data. You will calculate averages (means), medians, standard deviations, and ranges to get an overall picture of your data. For example, if you are tracking a client's pain levels over a period, you could calculate the average reduction in pain score between sessions.

How to do it:

- Calculate the mean (average), median, and mode to summarise the central tendency of your data.
- Use the standard deviation to measure the variability or spread of your data.

Time Series Analysis

If you are tracking changes over time—such as how a client's flexibility or swelling improves between treatment sessions—time series analysis can help you identify trends or patterns. This technique looks at how the data points change over a period, allowing you to see whether there's consistent progress or fluctuations.

How to do it:

- Plot your data over time (for example, using a graph or chart) and look for patterns or trends.
- You might notice that pain levels decrease steadily after each treatment session or that progress is inconsistent.

Comparative Analysis

If your case study involves multiple treatment approaches or clients, comparative analysis lets you compare different data sets. This technique is useful when you are trying to evaluate the effectiveness of two different treatment plans or modalities.

How to do it:

- Compare the average changes in outcomes (like pain levels or range of motion) between different treatments.

- Use statistical tests like t-tests* (inferential statistic) which are used to determine if there is a significant difference between the means of two groups and how they are relate, or ANOVA* (**AN**alysis **O**f **VA**riance) if you are comparing more than two groups to determine if the differences are statistically significant.

Let's say you are tracking a client's swelling reduction using a scale from 0 to 10. You measure this before each session and at the end of the course of treatment. After calculating the average pain reduction, you might notice that the average improvement is three points. This shows a significant reduction over time, confirming the effectiveness of your treatment plan.

*(T test is used to compare the means between two groups, whereas ANOVA is used to compare the means among three or more groups.)

Qualitative Data Analysis

Qualitative data is more subjective and descriptive. It is all about understanding the nuances of your client's experiences—such as feedback on how they feel, observations of their behaviour or posture, or emotional changes throughout treatment.

Key Techniques for Qualitative Data:

Thematic Analysis

Thematic analysis is a flexible method that helps you identify patterns or themes within qualitative data. If you have collected interview transcripts, open-ended survey responses, or observational notes, thematic analysis helps you categorise and make sense of these rich, descriptive data.

How to do it:

- Read your data and highlight recurring themes or patterns.
- Group similar responses or behaviours together to form themes (for example, increased comfort, better sleep, reduced stress).
- Look for trends or changes in the themes over time.

Content Analysis

Content analysis helps you analyse text (such as client feedback) by counting and categorising words or phrases. This is helpful if you have a lot of open-ended responses and want to identify which topics or feelings come up most often.

How to do it:

- Break down your data into manageable chunks, such as phrases or sentences.
- Count how often certain words or themes appear (for example, "relief," "pain," "stress reduction").
- Summarise the frequency of these terms and what they might indicate about the client's experience.

Narrative Analysis

Narrative analysis focuses on understanding the story behind your client's experience. This technique is particularly useful when you are looking at how the treatment process impacted your client over time, and how they view their journey.

How to do it:

- Review any narrative data (for example, client journaling, detailed case notes) and identify the stages of the client's treatment journey.
- Pay attention to how the client's story evolves—what changes do they note in their perspective, and how does the treatment fit into their overall narrative of healing?

Let's say your client mentioned that they felt "more energised" after a particular treatment. After analysing several client testimonials, you notice a common theme: clients are reporting an improvement in energy levels after certain modalities. You could interpret this as a positive outcome of your treatment plan, which helps reinforce the value of the techniques you are using.

Mixed-Methods Analysis

If you have collected both quantitative and qualitative data, a mixed-methods analysis combines the strengths of both. It is like having the best of both worlds, where the numbers provide the structure, and the qualitative insights add depth and understanding.

Key Techniques for Mixed-Methods:

Triangulation

Triangulation means using multiple sources or methods to validate your findings. This technique helps increase the credibility of your results by comparing data from different angles. For example, if your quantitative data shows a reduction in pain, but your qualitative data (client feedback) suggests an improvement in overall well-being, triangulation can help you integrate both findings into a more comprehensive conclusion.

How to do it:

- Cross-reference your quantitative findings with qualitative insights to check for consistency or patterns.
- If there are discrepancies, dive deeper into understanding why that might be.

Integration

Integration involves combining quantitative and qualitative data in a meaningful way. Instead of treating them separately, you merge the two to tell a complete story about your client's journey.

How to do it:

- Present both sets of data in the same analysis, showing how they complement each other.

  For example, you could compare the client's improvement in pain score (quantitative) with their feedback about feeling less stressed or more mobile (qualitative) to create a fuller picture of the outcome.

How to Visualise

Sometimes numbers and text alone do not tell the whole story. This is where visualisation comes in. Graphs, charts, and tables are fantastic tools to help make your data clearer and more digestible

Use **bar charts and line graphs** to show trends over time, like the reduction in swelling or improvement in flexibility.

Pie charts can be helpful for showing proportions, like the percentage of clients who report a particular improvement or symptom relief.

If you have a lot of data points, **tables** can help organise information neatly, allowing readers to compare data at a glance.

For example, you might track the client's range of motion before and after each treatment. A simple bar chart can show how the range of motion increases over time, making it easy to visualise progress.

Data analysis might seem daunting, but it is simply about interpreting the information you have collected and drawing meaningful insights from it. Whether you are dealing with numbers or stories, remember that your goal is to make the data work for you. It is not about complicated techniques but about using the right approach to get to the heart of what your client's journey has taught you.

So, play with the data, and let it tell you the story of how your treatment plans are making a difference.

Crunch the Numbers (and Stories)

Time to make sense of the data.

1. **Choose Your Method:** Are you analysing numbers, stories, or both? Write down your approach.
2. **Start with One Metric:** Focus on one key data point and begin your analysis.
3. **Summarise Your Findings:** Write a few sentences about what the data is telling you.

What patterns are you starting to notice?

Page left intentionally blank for your notes.

Interpreting Results

Now you have completed the hard work—gathered data, applied treatments, and kept track of every little detail along the way. Now comes the fun part: interpreting the results. This is where you take all that data, look for patterns, and figure out what it means in the context of your case study.

But interpreting results is not just about staring at numbers and seeing what pops up. It is about drawing conclusions that are meaningful, practical, and useful to your practice. Let's take a closer look at how to make sense of your findings and turn them into actionable insights.

Look for Patterns and Trends

This might sound obvious, but it is worth emphasising start by looking for trends in your data. Are there any patterns that stand out? For example, you might notice a consistent reduction in pain or swelling after each treatment session. Or maybe your client's mobility improves steadily, but at a slower pace.

You should look for the following:

- **Improvements or Deteriorations** - Has there been consistent progress in the outcomes you were tracking? If so, that is a good sign that your treatment plan is working. If there is little to no progress, it may suggest a need to reassess your approach.

- **Patterns Across Multiple Sessions** - Look at your data across different time points. Sometimes, changes might not be immediately visible, but over time, you might notice a clear upward or downward trend.

Example:

If you are tracking a client's range of motion, you might see that it improves after each treatment. But if the data shows a slight dip during certain sessions, it might indicate that those treatments need tweaking or that something else (like client compliance) could be impacting results.

Compare Results to Your Hypothesis or Goals

You need to revisit the objectives and goals you set at the beginning of the process. Were you expecting certain outcomes? Did your hypothesis hold up under scrutiny? You will want to compare your actual results to your initial expectations and see if they align.

You should consider the following:

- **Were your goals realistic?** - Did the improvements you tracked match what you thought was achievable? If your goals were too ambitious, it might explain why the results did not meet expectations.
- **Unexpected Findings –** Sometimes the results you get will not match what you anticipated. This can be a huge learning opportunity. Maybe your client experienced unexpected side effects, or you found a treatment modality that worked better than expected. Be open to adjusting your views based on what the data is telling you.

Example:

If your goal were to reduce swelling by 50 percent over six weeks and the actual reduction was 40 percent, this is still valuable information. It is not a failure—it is just an opportunity to refine your approach next time.

Assess the Significance of the Findings

This is where a bit of critical thinking comes into play. Are the results you are seeing practically or biologically significant or just a fluke?

Assessing the significance of your findings is a crucial step in completing your case study. This is where you reflect on what your results mean in the context of your research question, client outcomes, and the broader field of massage therapy. You should start by identifying the key outcomes of your study and consider how they compare to your initial objectives. Did you achieve the results you expected, or were there any surprises along the way? By understanding these outcomes, it will help you gauge the overall success of your intervention or observation.

Next, consider how your findings contribute to the existing body of knowledge. Do they confirm, challenge, or expand upon previous research or accepted practices? When you highlight these connections it not only strengthens the credibility of your study but also situates it within the larger professional conversation. Additionally, you should reflect on any limitations or challenges you have encountered during your study. Were there factors that may have influenced the results, such as sample size, client compliance, or external variables?

Finally, think about the practical implications of your findings. How can they be applied in a real-world massage therapy setting? Could your insights help other therapists refine their techniques, improve client outcomes, or address specific challenges in their practice? By thoughtfully assessing the significance of your findings, you ensure that your case study has lasting value and relevance.

While you may not be running formal studies with large sample sizes, it is still important to understand whether your findings are likely to hold up beyond the specific client you are studying.

Following are some questions you may want to ask:

What is the margin of error?

Is there a chance that what you are seeing is simply due to random variation or external factors? A client's improvement might be influenced by factors other than your treatments—like changes in lifestyle, stress levels, or even placebo effects.

Can the results be generalised?

If your case study is based on a single client, remember that the results might not apply to everyone. However, you can still draw conclusions that are valuable in the context of your own practice.

Say you are tracking pain reduction for a client, and the results show a significant decrease in their pain levels. Before you assume this outcome can be replicated with every client, ask yourself whether any external factors (like medication changes or other therapies they might have undergone) could have influenced the result.

Link the Results to the Treatment Plan

When interpreting results, always link them back to your treatment plan. Did the techniques you used have the desired effect? Or were there any modifications that you wish you had made earlier? This step helps you evaluate the effectiveness of your treatments and refine your methods.

Look at the data and see if some treatments led to more significant improvements than others. For instance, if certain modalities seem to work better for pain relief, those could be the treatments you prioritise in future case studies or client treatments.

Did the treatment duration align with the expected outcomes? If your client's improvement plateaued early, maybe they needed longer treatment periods or more frequent sessions.

If you used a combination of massage techniques and lymphatic drainage, and your client's swelling reduced significantly, you might conclude that these treatments were most effective. But if you notice that a specific technique (such as deep tissue massage) did not yield much progress, you could decide to minimise its use in the future.

Contextualise the Results

Interpreting results is not just about what the data shows—it is about what the data means in the context of the whole case study. Your client's progress is influenced by many factors, including their lifestyle, compliance with the treatment plan, and even their psychological state. Be sure to consider the bigger picture when interpreting your results.

Did your client have other health issues or environmental factors that could have influenced their outcomes? For example, if they were stressed or had a poor diet, it could impact their recovery, and this should be factored into your interpretation.

How does your client feel about the results? Sometimes, the numbers might not tell the whole story. If a client reports feeling better, even if the physical changes are subtle, this could still indicate success in your approach.

If your client reports feeling "more relaxed" or "less stressed" even when the data shows only a slight improvement in swelling or pain, it suggests that the psychological benefits of treatment (like stress reduction or relaxation) might be contributing to their overall well-being.

Draw Conclusions and Make Recommendations

Now that you have analysed your results and considered the broader context, it is time to draw your conclusions. What can you say about the effectiveness of your treatment plan? Did it work as expected? And if not, what changes would you recommend for future cases?

What to Consider:

- **Effectiveness:**
  Can you confidently say your treatment plan worked? If so, what aspects of the plan would you continue to use with other clients?

- **Improvements for Future Treatments:** If the results were not exactly what you expected, what could be improved next time? You may need to adjust treatment techniques, frequency, or even the way you engage with the client to encourage better results.

If your case study shows moderate success with your treatment plan, your conclusion might be something like: "The treatment plan effectively reduced swelling and pain, but additional sessions or a modified approach may be necessary for longer-lasting results."

Interpreting results is more than just a numbers game—it is about making sense of the data and drawing practical conclusions that will benefit your practice. Think of it as solving a puzzle: each piece of data contributes to the bigger picture of your client's journey. So, take your time, look for patterns, and always remember that even unexpected results offer valuable insights. By refining your approach based on what you learn, you will be better equipped to achieve even better outcomes for your clients in the future.

Making Sense of It All

Let's draw some meaningful conclusions.

1. **Summarise Your Findings:** Write down the key outcomes in plain language.
2. **Compare to Objectives:** Did you the results support your original hypothesis? Why or why not?
3. **Identify Key Takeaways:** List 2–3 big insights from your study.

What is the most valuable lesson from your findings?

Page left intentionally blank for your notes.

Structuring Your Report

Now that you have gathered your data, monitored progress, and interpreted the results, it is time to bring everything together into a report. Writing a case study is about presenting your findings in a clear, concise, and structured way. It is about showing what you did and what happened, telling the story of your client's journey, the treatment process, and how your approach helped (or did not help) them.

A well-structured report will help you convey your insights effectively, whether you are presenting it to a peer, a supervisor, or even yourself for future reference. Let's break it down, step by step, to ensure you cover all the bases.

Title Page

The title page is the first impression your report will make, so keep it clean and professional. Include:

Title of the Case Study

Make it descriptive but concise. It should give readers a clear idea of what your case study is about. For example, "Treatment of Chronic Shoulder Pain Through Manual Therapy" or "A Case Study on Lymphatic Drainage for Post-Surgical Swelling."

Your Name and Qualifications

This gives credibility to your work. Include your name, credentials, and any relevant qualifications that tie into the case study (for example, certified remedial massage therapist, lymphatic therapy specialist).

Date

The date the case study is being presented or submitted.

Key Words

Including keywords under the title of a case study is essential for increasing its visibility and accessibility in academic and professional databases. Keywords help researchers, practitioners, and publishers quickly identify the study's focus, ensuring it reaches the right audience. They also improve searchability in journal indexes, databases like PubMed and Google Scholar, and even general search engines. Well-chosen keywords enhance the impact of the case study by making it easier to find, reference, and apply in relevant clinical or research settings.

Abstract (Optional, but Recommended)

An abstract is a brief summary of the entire report. It should give the reader a snapshot of the problem, treatment methods, and key findings. While it is optional, an abstract can be useful for busy readers who just want to get the gist of the study before diving into the details.

A good abstract should be about 150-250 words and briefly cover:

- The client's issue (for example, "Chronic neck pain after a car accident")
- The treatment methods used (For example, "Massage therapy, myofascial release, and stretching")
- The key results (For example, "Reduction in pain intensity and improved range of motion")
- Any conclusions or recommendations.

Introduction

Here is where you set the scene for your readers. The introduction should give enough background information, so the reader understands the context of the case study. Answer the following:

Client Background

Provide a brief overview of the client (respecting confidentiality, of course). Who are they (age, occupation, medical history)? What was their initial complaint or concern? This helps the reader understand the scope of the case.

Problem Statement

What issue are you trying to address with your treatment? Be clear about the symptoms or condition the client is experiencing and why it is relevant to study.

Objective of the Case Study

What was the goal of your case study? Were you trying to test a specific treatment technique or track the progress of a particular condition? Outline the objectives in a sentence or two.

Literature Review (Optional, but Valuable)

This section ties your case study into the broader field of practice. You do not have to go too deep, but it is important to show that you have considered existing research or expert opinions in your approach.

Relevant Research or Theories

Are there any studies or theories that support your treatment approach? Briefly mention any relevant findings that justify why you chose the treatment plan you did.

Knowledge Gaps or Controversies

If applicable, highlight any gaps in existing knowledge or controversies that your case study might help clarify. For instance, if there's debate about a specific massage technique, you can note how your case study might contribute to the ongoing discussion.

Methodology

This is where you outline how you approached the case study. You are giving your readers a roadmap of what you did and how you did it, so they can understand your approach and evaluate the validity of your findings.

Client Assessment

Briefly summarise the assessment process. What was your initial evaluation of the client's condition? Include any tools or techniques you used (For example, range of motion testing, visual assessments).

Treatment Plan

Describe the treatments you implemented. Be specific about the techniques used (For example, Swedish massage, deep tissue, lymphatic drainage) and the duration/frequency of the treatments.

Data Collection

How did you track the client's progress? Did you use objective measurements (For example, pain scale, swelling reduction) or subjective ones (For example, client feedback)?

Results

Now we get to the heart of the report: the results. This is where you will present the findings from your case study in a clear and logical manner.

Data Presentation

Present the data in a way that is easy to digest—charts, photographs, tables, or graphs work well here. Use visuals to highlight key progress points, like pain reduction or improved mobility.

Analysis

Analyse the data and highlight trends or key moments of improvement (or lack thereof). Do not just present the numbers—interpret them and tie them back to the treatment you provided.

Discussion

In the discussion section, you will take a deeper dive into your results and provide a thoughtful interpretation. Here, you will discuss the implications of your findings, any unexpected outcomes, and how your approach could be applied or modified in future cases.

What Worked

Which parts of your treatment plan were most effective? Was there a specific technique that produced noticeable results?

What Could Be Improved

Were there any aspects of the treatment that did not work as well as expected? Did you learn anything from the experience that would change your approach in future case studies?

Comparison to Existing Literature

If you referenced studies or theories earlier, this is where you can compare your results to what has already been published. Did your findings align with existing research?

Conclusion

The conclusion is your opportunity to wrap everything up neatly. Summarise the key points from your case study and highlight the most important takeaway for your readers. Your conclusion should be concise and to the point, leaving the reader with a clear understanding of what you have learned and how it might apply in a broader context.

Summary of Key Findings

Restate your most important conclusions in a few sentences. What were the main takeaways from your case study?

Implications for Future Practice

How might this case study influence your approach to treating similar clients in the future? What could other therapists learn from your experience?

Suggestions for Further Research or Practice

If applicable, suggest areas where further research is needed or where your case study could be expanded upon.

References

If you have cited any research, articles, or other resources, this is where you will list them. Make sure to follow the appropriate citation style (APA, MLA, etc.) and include all the details—author, title, publication date, and source.

Appendices (If Necessary)

If there is any supplementary information you think is important but too detailed for the main sections of your report, include it in the appendices. This could include:

- Client Consent Forms
- Detailed Assessment Tools
- Additional Data or Charts
- Photographs (with proper consent)

A well-structured case study report is like telling a story. You guide your reader from beginning to end, showing them what your client went through, what treatment was applied, and the results that followed. The clearer and more organised you are, the easier it will be for others to learn from your experience and apply those lessons in their own practices. Remember: this report is not just about showing what you did—it is about making your findings meaningful and applicable for future clients and case studies.

Time to Bring It All Together

Drafting the report might feel like a big task, but let's break it down into bite-sized pieces.

1. **Outline Your Report:** Write down the main sections you will include (For example, Introduction, Objectives, Methods, Results, Conclusion).
2. **Draft the Introduction:** Write 2–3 sentences explaining *why* you conducted this case study and *what* you aimed to achieve.
3. **Sketch Out the Flow:** Create a rough flowchart showing how your report will progress from one section to the next.

If someone only read your introduction, would they understand what your study is about?

Page left intentionally blank for your notes.

Using Visual Aids

When it comes to writing a case study, the power of visuals cannot be overstated. They are not just there to make your report look pretty—they are there to help tell the story, clarify complex information, and make your findings easier to understand. Whether you are showing client progress, illustrating treatment methods, or presenting data, visuals can make all the difference. Let's talk about how and why you should incorporate visual aids into your case study.

Why Use Visual Aids?

This section discussed why visuals are so effective. Humans are wired to process images faster than text. Our brains can process images in a fraction of a second, and when you use visuals in your case study, they can help:

- **Enhance Understanding:** Visuals make data easier to digest, turning abstract concepts into something concrete.

- **Clarify Findings:** Sometimes numbers and statistics can be overwhelming. Graphs and charts simplify those findings, making it easier for readers to see trends or progress.

- **Engage the Reader:** A case study full of text can be overwhelming, but visuals break things up and keep readers engaged. They draw attention, highlight key points, and keep the focus on essential information.

Types of Visual Aids to Include

There are several types of visuals you can use in your case study. Let's go over a few that will help you tell your story in a clear and engaging way.

Client Photos or Diagrams

Photographs and diagrams can be extremely helpful for showing the client's condition at various stages. They give readers a visual representation of progress over time, especially if you are treating visible conditions like swelling, bruising, or muscle tension.

First, a big rule—**always** get written consent from your client before using any photos. Respect their privacy and ensure that they understand how the photos will be used. See the section on Client Consent for more information.

You can use photographs such as before-and-after images, progress photos showing changes in posture, range of motion, or swelling, or any other visible condition to show real-world results. You can also use diagrams to show areas of tension or pain during your assessment.

Place the images in relevant sections of your report, such as the introduction (for initial assessment photos) and the results (for progress pictures).

The following photo example shows the initial assessment photo on the left and the results photo on the right.

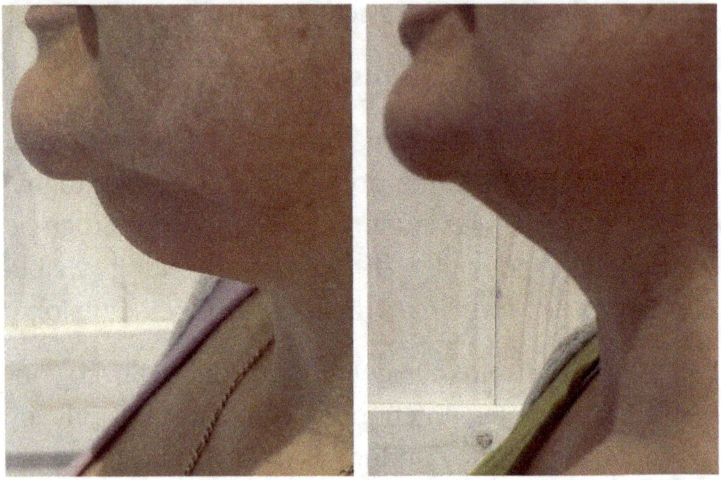

Graphs and Charts

When you are dealing with data, graphs and charts are invaluable. They help you display information clearly and concisely. They are especially useful for illustrating changes over time or comparing data points.

Following are types of graphs to consider:

- **Bar charts** for comparing measurements like pain levels, range of motion, or swelling at different points in the treatment plan.

- **Line graphs** for showing changes over time, such as progress in symptom reduction over several sessions.

- **Pie charts** for demonstrating distribution or proportions, like client feedback (For example, satisfaction levels or symptom improvement).

Include graphs when you are presenting quantitative data like pain scales or improvement percentages. Make sure to label everything clearly so readers can easily interpret the data.

The following example illustrates the use of a graph showing changes in various leg parts at various sessions:

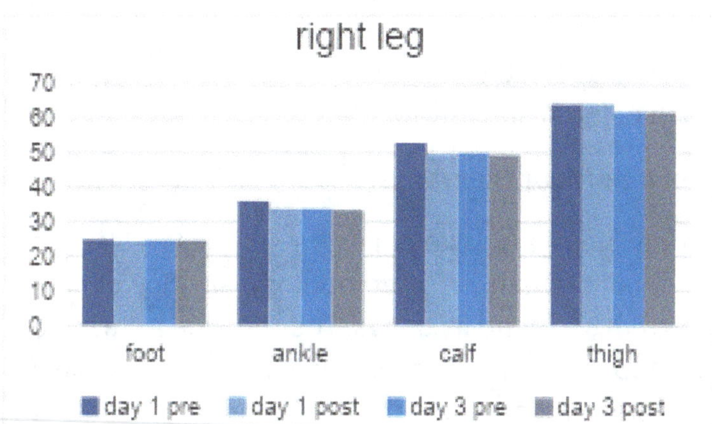

Tables

Tables help to organise and present data in a simple, easy-to-read format. If you have multiple data points to compare (for example, assessment results, treatment methods, and progress), a table is an excellent choice.

Include the following information in a table:

- **Assessment results** before and after treatment
- **Treatment sessions** with details (date, techniques used, client feedback, etc.)
- **Measurement data** (pain levels, range of motion, etc.)

Keep tables clean and organised with clear headers. Do not overcrowd them—only include relevant data that will add value to your report. Make sure you label each column and row for clarity.

Flowcharts or Diagrams

When you are explaining a process—like your treatment plan or methodology—a flowchart or diagram can simplify things. They provide a clear step-by-step view of what you did, which makes it easier for readers to follow your logic and approach.

You can use flowcharts to outline your treatment approach or how you analysed client data. Diagrams can be useful when showing how different treatment techniques relate to the problem.

Keep flowcharts simple and easy to follow, with arrows that clearly indicate the direction of your process. Use short, descriptive phrases to avoid overcrowding the diagram.

Client Feedback Quotes

Sometimes, the most powerful visuals are not pictures or graphs—they are words. Client testimonials or direct feedback quotes add a human touch to your case study, offering insights into their personal experience with your treatment.

Include key quotes from your client that highlight their feelings about the treatment process or the results. These testimonials can help add depth to your case study and show the emotional or personal impact of your work.

Sprinkle these quotes throughout your report, especially in the “Results” or “Discussion” sections, to add a personal dimension to the more technical data.

Best Practices for Using Visual Aids

This section outlines how to effectively use visuals aids in your case study.

Keep It Simple

Visuals aids should simplify information, not overwhelm the reader. Avoid cluttering your report with too many visuals aids or overly complex charts. Choose the ones that best support your point, and make sure each one has a clear purpose.

Be Clear and Consistent

Always label your visual aids clearly. This includes:

- **Titles or captions** explaining what the visual represents.
- **Labels** for axes in graphs or measurements in tables.
- **Legends** for charts that explain what different colours or symbols represent.

Also, try to maintain a consistent style throughout your case study. Use similar colours, fonts, and layouts to ensure your report feels cohesive.

Focus on Quality, Not Quantity

It is tempting to throw in a lot of visuals to “spice up” your report, but quality matters more than quantity. Only include visual aids that add value to your case study. A few well-chosen, high-quality images or charts can be far more effective than a dozen irrelevant ones.

Explain the Visuals

Just adding visuals is not enough. You need to explain what each one represents and how it supports your findings. Be sure to reference each visual in the body of your text, pointing out key observations and drawing conclusions from the data.

Respect Client Privacy

If you are using client photos, feedback, or any personal data, it is critically important that you ensure that you have written consent and are abiding by confidentiality agreements. Always protect your clients’ privacy and be transparent about how their information will be used.

Visual aids are more than just decoration—they are essential tools for helping your readers understand your case study. When used properly, they make your findings clearer, more engaging, and easier to interpret. By using a variety of visuals (photos, graphs, charts, tables, and feedback quotes) and following best practices for clarity and consistency, you will ensure that your case study is not only informative but also a pleasure to read. So, next time you are writing up your case study, remember: the right visual aid at the right moment can make all the difference in how your story is told.

Make Your Report Pop

Visual aids are not just for decoration—they tell a story.

1. **Choose Your Visuals:** Decide which charts, graphs, or photos best represent your findings.
2. **Create One Visual Aid:** Build one visual aid (for example, a simple chart showing progress over time).
3. **Add Context:** Write a caption explaining *what* the visual shows and *why* it matters.

Does your visual aid clarify your findings, or does it raise more questions?

Page left intentionally blank for your notes.

Sharing and Utilising Case Studies

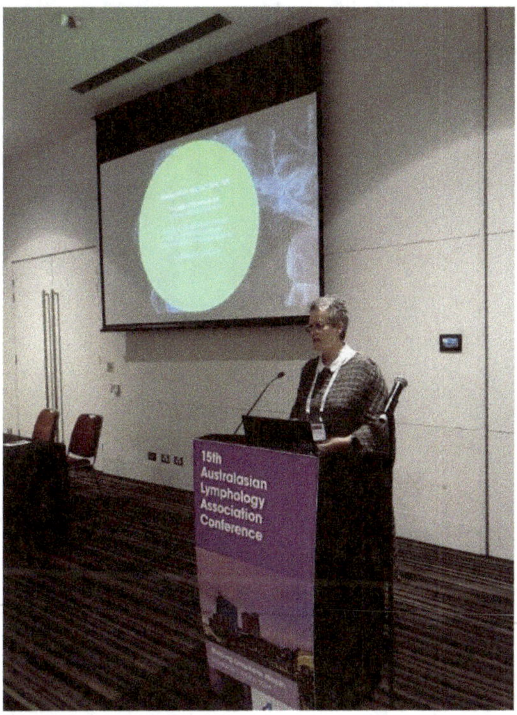

Congratulations on completing your case study! What a huge effort! It is time to share your case study with the world. Publishing your case study is not just about getting your findings out there; it is also about establishing yourself as someone who contributes to the profession and offers valuable insights. But where should you publish it, and how can you make sure the right people see it?

Choose the Right Platform for Publishing

The first thing you need to consider is where you want to publish your case study. There are so many options out there, and each platform has its own set of benefits and challenges. Following are a few to consider:

Academic Journals

If your case study has a strong research component or you are looking to make a serious academic contribution, you should consider academic journals. These are typically peer-reviewed, which adds a layer of credibility to your work.

- **Pros:**
  - Professional recognition
  - Peer validation from other experts in your field
  - It can really help your professional reputation.
- **Cons:**
  - It can take several months to be published

- There are often strict guidelines and formatting rules for publication
- You will need solid research to meet their standards.

Start by finding journals that specialise in massage therapy, healthcare, or whatever niche your case study fits into. Be sure to read their submission guidelines closely. Different Journals may require specific formatting and reference style, but they will inform you of what they require, if what you have submitted needs editing.

Industry-Specific Websites or Blogs

If you are more interested in sharing your case study with fellow professionals in the massage therapy community, industry websites or blogs might be your best platform for sharing. These platforms are often looking for real-world examples that can help others improve their practice.

- **Pros:**
    - You will reach a specific, engaged audience.
    - You can see your case study published much faster.
    - It helps you connect with others in your field.
- **Cons:**
    - It is not as prestigious as an academic journal (but that does not mean it is not valuable!)
    - You might not reach an audience outside of your industry.

Look for guest post opportunities on websites, blogs, or forums related to your field. Many industry websites are open to guest contributions, so just check their submission guidelines and pitch your case study!

Conferences

If you have presented your case study (poster presentation or podium presentation) at a conference (or plan to), you might be able to have it published in the conference proceedings. This is a great way to share your work with people who are already invested in your field.

- **Pros:**
    - The audience is already interested in your area of expertise.
    - It is great opportunity for networking and professional development.
- **Cons:**
    - Your audience is limited to conference attendees.
    - It might not get as much attention outside of the event.

Check with the conference organisers to see if they offer an opportunity to have your case study published as part of their proceedings. It is often a nice bonus to presenting, and it can help your work get noticed within that community.

Self-Publishing (Books or E-books)

If you have a lot to say, or you want to turn your case study into a more comprehensive guide, you may want to consider self-publishing. Whether as an e-book or printed book, you will have full control over the content, style, and distribution.

- **Pros:**
    - You control everything—content, format, and pricing.
    - It is an easy way to reach a global audience through various distribution platforms.
    - You can establish yourself as a thought leader.
- **Cons:**
    - You are responsible for everything—writing, design, editing, marketing, and more.
    - You will need to market the book to ensure it gets noticed.
    - There is a bit more upfront work (but it can be extremely rewarding!)

Big-name publishing platforms make it easy (albeit expensive) to publish an e-book or paperback. If you are self-publishing a collection of case studies, make sure to format it properly so it is reader-friendly and professional-looking.

Social Media and Professional Networks

For a more informal, quicker way to get your case study out there, social media and professional networks are a great option. You can share snippets of your case study, or link to a full version hosted on your website or blog.

- **Pros:**
    - Instant feedback and engagement from your network
    - You can build your professional brand.
    - You can promote it for free!
- **Cons:**
    - It is not as formal or academically recognised.
    - It can get lost in the noise of your followers' feeds.

You can post summaries, insights, or even images related to your case study on social media. If you have a blog, link back to the full version of your case study there. If you are in professional groups, consider sharing your work there too!

Prepare Your Case Study for Publication

Now that you have chosen where to publish, it is time to make sure your case study is ready for the spotlight. Here is a checklist to help you prepare:

Clarity and Precision

Make sure your case study is easy to follow and understand. Avoid jargon unless it is necessary, and do not forget to break things down with visual aids. People learn better when they can see things as well as read about them.

Double-Check Ethical Considerations

Have you obtained consent from your client? Is the client safe? Are all identifying details kept confidential? If you are using photos, have you made sure you have permission? Always make sure you are ethical in your approach—this is key.

Follow Submission Guidelines

Different platforms have different rules. Whether it is an academic journal or a blog, make sure you know their specific requirements, like word count, formatting, and citation style.

Proofread and Edit

Typos are never fun. Before submitting, give your work a once-over (or even a second or third look!) to ensure it is polished. You might even want to ask a colleague to read it and give feedback.

Provide Supplementary Materials

If your platform requests any additional resources (like treatment plans or forms), have those ready to go. They can make your case study more robust and useful to others.

Promote Your Case Study

Once your case study is published, the job is not over. Take this time to get the word out and make sure people see it! Here are some ideas for promoting it:

Share on social media

Post about your case study on all your platforms. Invite your followers to read, comment, and share it with their networks.

Share with Your Professional Network

Ask colleagues, clients, or anyone who might benefit from your case study to read it and share it with their contacts.

Engage in Online Discussions

Join Facebook groups, LinkedIn communities, or other online forums in your field. Share your case study when relevant and offer to discuss it with others.

Start a Blog or Newsletter

If you have a blog or mailing list, share a brief summary of your case study with a link to the full version. It is a fantastic way to keep your audience updated and engaged with your work.

Publishing your case study is important—it is your chance to show what you have learned, contribute to your profession, and get your name out there as a professional. Whether you choose to go the academic route, self-publish a book, or post on social media, make sure you are prepared and that your work is ethical and well-presented. And remember, once it is published, do not just let it sit there—promote it, share it, and engage with others to get the most out of your hard work!

Share Your Hard Work

1. **Identify Your Platform:** Write down 1–2 potential places to publish your case study (for example, journals, association newsletters, etc.).

2. **Check Submission Guidelines:** Look up the requirements for one platform and jot down the key points.

3. **Write a Summary Abstract:** Craft a 3–4 sentence summary of your case study that highlights the most important findings.

What impact do you hope your published case study will have on the profession?

Page left intentionally blank for your notes.

Presenting your Findings

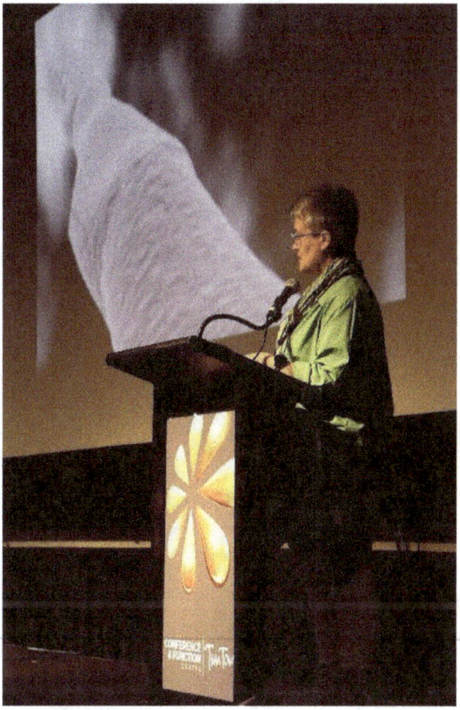

All right, now that you have done the challenging work of gathering data, conducting your study, and publishing your case study, you should consider presenting your findings to an audience. This is where you get to shine and really communicate the value of your work to others. Presenting your findings is not just about sharing your results; it is about telling a story in a way that is clear, engaging, and informative. So, let's walk through some key points to help you present your findings in the best way possible.

Know Your Audience

Before you start presenting, it is essential to know who your audience is. Are you presenting to a group of fellow massage therapists, academic researchers, or a broader healthcare audience? The way you present your findings will differ based on who you are speaking to.

If Your Audience Is Fellow Practitioners

You will want to focus on practical implications. Show them how your case study can directly impact their practice, improve outcomes, or inspire novel approaches. You should tailor your language so that is is familiar to them and consider their day-to-day challenges.

If Your Audience Is Academics or Researchers

Emphasise the scientific and methodological rigor of your study. Discuss your research methods in detail, address any limitations, and present your findings through data and analysis.

If Your Audience Is a Broader Healthcare Group

Strike a balance between accessibility and professionalism. You may need to provide some background context to ensure they understand the scope and relevance of your study. Keep it engaging but informative and avoid overwhelming them with technical details unless necessary.

Organise Your Presentation

Good organisation is key when presenting your findings. It helps your audience follow your narrative, understand your results, and engage with the content.

Following is a simple structure to keep things flowing:

Start with the Background

Give your audience context for the case study. Why did you choose this particular case? What problem were you addressing? This sets the stage for understanding the significance of your findings.

State Your Objectives

What were you trying to achieve with the case study? Were you testing a specific treatment, exploring a new technique, or looking for trends? Clearly outline your goals so your audience knows what to expect.

Present Your Methodology

Discuss how you gathered your data. Explain your assessment process, treatment plan, and monitoring strategies. Remember to keep it understandable and not overly technical (unless it is necessary for your audience).

Share Your Results

Now, the fun part! Present your findings clearly and logically. Use visual aids from your case study to help tell the story because they can make your results more compelling and easier to understand.

Discuss the Implications

What do your results mean for your practice or your field? How can others apply your findings in their own work? This is where you connect the dots for your audience and show them why your case study matters.

Addressing questions from the Audience

Summarise the main points of your presentation. Highlight the key lessons, the success of your approach, and any challenges you faced. Leave your audience with something to think about and a clear understanding of how to apply your findings.

Use Visual Aids Effectively

Humans are visual creatures, and we retain information better when it is presented with the right visuals. This is where photos, graphs, and charts come into play. But be mindful—your visuals should complement and clarify your findings, not overwhelm them.

Use Before-and-After Photos (If Applicable)

Photos can be particularly powerful in massage therapy case studies, especially if you are showing how a treatment improved a client's condition. Just be sure you have proper consent from your client before you share any photos publicly.

Incorporate Charts and Graphs

For more quantitative case studies, graphs are a great way to show trends, improvements, or changes over time. Whether it is tracking pain levels, range of motion, or progress towards treatment goals, a good graph can really make your results pop.

Use Simple Diagrams or Flowcharts

These can be helpful to show processes, treatment plans, or progress tracking in a way that is easy for your audience to follow.

Avoid Overloading with Text

Too much text can make your presentation feel like a lecture. Use bullet points and concise statements to highlight key ideas. Your visuals should carry the weight of your findings.

Engage Your Audience

Presenting findings is not a one-way street. You want to engage your audience and invite discussion. Here are some ways to do that:

Ask Questions

Pose thought-provoking questions throughout your presentation to get your audience thinking. You could ask something like, “Has anyone else tried this technique in their practice?” or “What would you do differently based on these results?”

Encourage Feedback

Be open to feedback, whether positive or constructive. Asking for feedback can help you refine your approach in future case studies and can foster valuable professional connections.

Use Real-Life Examples

People love stories! If possible, share anecdotes or specific experiences that highlight your results. This makes your case study more relatable and memorable for your audience. Be mindful to maintain client privacy and confidentiality.

Practice Your Delivery

The best case study in the world can fall flat if the delivery is not engaging. Practice, practice, practice. Here are a few tips:

Know Your Material

You do not want to sound like you are reading off a script, so make sure you know your case study inside and out. This will help you speak confidently and naturally.

Be Clear and Concise

Stick to the main points. If you are giving a presentation with a time limit, make sure you stay on track and cover the most important aspects of your case study.

Be Passionate

Show your audience why you are excited about your findings! If you believe in your work, your passion will shine through and keep them engaged.

Conclude with Actionable Takeaways

When you wrap up, make sure your audience leaves with actionable takeaways. What can they learn from your case study, and how can they apply it to their own work? Whether it is a new treatment approach, a different way of tracking progress, or an insight into client care, the goal is to offer something practical and valuable.

Handling Questions

Lastly, be prepared for questions. After your presentation, open the floor for discussion, but do not be caught off guard. Here is how you can handle questions:

Be Honest

If you do not have an answer to a question, it is okay to admit it. Offer to follow up after the presentation or to refer to additional resources.

Encourage Dialogue

Do not just give a one-word answer. Engage with the question and offer your perspective on it.

Stay calm

If someone asks a difficult question: acknowledge this, breathe, and take your time to answer. Being calm and present will allow you time enough to answer. Doing this will calm you and reassure your audience that you know what you are talking about.

Presenting your findings is the ultimate step in sharing the fruits of your hard work. By knowing your audience, structuring your presentation effectively, using visuals to support your results, and engaging with your audience, you can make a powerful impact. The key is to be clear, concise, and confident—so your findings are both informative and memorable. Remember, your case study has the potential to inspire others, so make sure you give it the attention it deserves in your presentation.

Take the Stage (or the Screen)

Whether it is at a conference or an online webinar, let's get presentation-ready.

1. **Create a Presentation Outline:** Write down 4–5 main points you will cover when sharing your case study.
2. **Prepare a Key Slide:** Create one slide that summarises your most important finding.
3. **Practice Your Opening Statement:** Write and rehearse the first 30 seconds of your presentation.

What is one story or insight from your case study that would really grab your audience's attention?

Let your case study participants know that they may be able to also be part of the presentation or publication of your findings - if they want to. Most might want to remain anonymous, but some may like the idea of being fully involved.

Page left intentionally blank for your notes

Applying Case Study Insights

Now that you have gone through the process of collecting data, analysing it, presenting your findings, and even publishing your case study, it is time to ask: "What's next?" Applying the insights from your case study is where the real magic happens. These insights do not just sit on a shelf—they can actively enhance your practice, inform future treatment plans, and even influence how you approach client care moving forward.

Let's dive into how you can apply the lessons you have learned from your case study to level up your practice and make a meaningful impact on your clients.

Refine Treatment Techniques

One of the most immediate ways to apply your case study insights is to fine-tune your treatment techniques. If your case study has revealed that a specific approach works exceptionally well for certain conditions, it is time to incorporate that technique more deliberately into your practice.

Identify Patterns and Trends

Look for patterns in your results. For example, if you noticed significant improvement in your client's condition with a combination of techniques—say, deep tissue massage and lymphatic drainage—consider using this as your go-to approach for similar cases in the future.

Test and Adapt

A case study is an experiment, and applying its insights is a bit like testing a hypothesis. Use what you have learned, but do not be afraid to tweak things based on how future clients respond. It is all about refining and improving your practice over time.

Share Insights with Colleagues

If you have found a treatment technique that yields impressive results, share it with your colleagues or mentors. A fresh perspective could help you refine your approach even further, and you might be able to collaborate on developing a new technique that could benefit others in the field.

Enhance Client Communication

Another way to apply case study insights is by improving the way you communicate with clients. After all, the success of a treatment plan is not just about the techniques you use; it is also about how well you work with your clients to set expectations, track progress, and build trust.

Tailor Your Approach to Individual Clients

What did you learn about your client's unique needs from your case study? Maybe your study revealed the importance of personalised care plans that consider specific lifestyle factors. Now, you can apply that insight by tailoring your client assessments and treatment strategies to be more individualised and responsive to each person's situation.

Build Better Client Relationships

Your case study probably highlighted areas where communication with your client made a difference, whether it was explaining the treatment process, setting clear expectations, or providing emotional support. Moving forward, use those insights to improve how you relate to clients on an individual level, fostering trust and collaboration.

Use Data to Drive Conversations

If you tracked metrics in your case study (like pain levels, range of motion, or other progress indicators), bring that data into your client discussions. By showing your clients the tangible evidence of their progress you can reinforce their commitment to treatment and keep them motivated.

Improving Your Practice

The insights from your case study can also be used to improve the overall effectiveness of your practice, both in terms of treatment outcomes and operational efficiency.

Review Your Client Intake Process

If your case study revealed that certain assessments or questions led to better outcomes, consider revising your client intake form or initial consultation process. A more detailed lifestyle questionnaire would give you insights into factors that impact your clients' recovery or treatment results. Use the data to inform your intake procedures.

Streamline Your Treatment Plans

From your case study, you might have found that certain treatment approaches work better for particular conditions or types of clients. Use this information to create a streamlined approach for managing similar cases in the future, which will save you time and increase the effectiveness of your treatment protocols.

Develop New Protocols

If your case study gave you new insights into how specific treatments or techniques affected your clients, use that knowledge to develop new practice protocols or even offer new services. For example, if your study showed how a combination of massage therapy and stretches provided optimal results, create a protocol for future clients based on these findings.

Educate Clients and Other Professionals

You have gathered valuable information through your case study, and it is important to share that knowledge—not just for the sake of your own practice, but to contribute to the wider massage therapy community.

Client Education

Do not keep your insights to yourself! Educate your clients on the benefits of the techniques or approaches that worked well in your case study. This can help clients understand how and why certain treatments will help them and empower them to take more control over their own health journey.

Share with Fellow Practitioners

If your case study revealed new or effective treatment techniques, share your findings with your colleagues, whether that is through informal chats, workshops, or formal presentations. Sharing knowledge can spark valuable discussions and may even lead to collaborative efforts to develop new practices within your field.

Create Educational Resources

Consider turning your case study findings into helpful resources for your clients or fellow therapists. This could be a handout, an instructional video, or even a blog post that outlines the key lessons you have learned and how others can benefit from them.

Contribute to Research and Advance the Field

Beyond your individual practice, the insights you have gathered can contribute to advancing the massage therapy field. When you apply your findings through formal channels like research publications, industry discussions, or workshops it can help push the boundaries of what is known about effective massage therapy practices.

Presenting at Conferences

If your case study is particularly innovative or has yielded important insights, consider presenting your findings at a professional conference or seminar. This not only helps raise your profile as an expert in your field but also contributes to the ongoing development of massage therapy practices.

Publishing Your Work

You can also publish your case study in professional journals, newsletters, or even on social media to share your findings with a larger audience. This can help others learn from your work, contribute to the evidence base for massage therapy, and inspire new research or case studies in the field.

Advocacy for Best Practices

As you apply your case study insights in your own practice, you will likely develop a deeper understanding of best practices in the field. Use that knowledge to advocate for better standards of care, improved techniques, or more evidence-based approaches in massage therapy.

Applying the insights from your case study is where the real value lies. It is not just about collecting data and publishing your findings—it is about using what you have learned to improve your practice, help your clients, and contribute to the broader massage therapy community. Whether you are refining your treatment techniques, improving client communication, or sharing your findings with others, the goal is to turn your case study into actionable change. So, take those lessons, apply them, and keep growing—because the work does not end when the case study is finished; it is just the beginning.

For me personally, conducting case studies and applying the insights I gained from them has had a transformative impact on my professional journey. The results of my own case studies did not just stay within the walls of my practice—they opened doors for me. They led to me being invited as a speaker at industry conferences, where I could share my findings and discuss best practices with my peers. It was through these experiences that I was inspired to create a course on case studies for massage therapists and write this book. The power of case studies has not only deepened my understanding of the craft but has also enabled me to contribute to the wider community by educating others and advocating for better practices across the profession.

From Insights to Action

Make sure your findings do not just sit on a shelf!

1. **Identify Practical Applications:** Write down 2–3 ways your findings can be applied in your own practice.
2. **Share with a Colleague:** Talk to another therapist about your findings and get their perspective.
3. **Write a Quick Tip:** Draft one actionable tip based on your findings that other therapists could use immediately.

What is one small change you have already made in your practice because of this study?

Page left intentionally blank for your notes

Incorporating Feedback

Once you have completed your case study, the work does not end there. In fact, one of the most valuable steps you can take is to gather and incorporate feedback. Feedback is not just about spotting mistakes or areas that need improvement—it is a tool for growth, refinement, and ensuring that your approach is as effective as possible.

Let's talk about why feedback matters and how you can effectively use it to enhance your case study and elevate your practice.

Why Feedback Matters

Feedback, whether it comes from clients, colleagues, mentors, or even your own self-reflection, is an essential part of improving your work. In the context of case studies, it helps you see things from a fresh perspective, points out areas that could be clearer or more precise, and allows you to refine your methods for future cases.

Objective Evaluation

Sometimes, when you are deeply involved in a project, it is hard to see clearly through the detail. Feedback provides an objective set of eyes that can point out blind spots, areas where something is not as clear as it could be, or where you may have missed an important piece of the puzzle.

Builds Confidence

Receiving positive feedback reassures you that you are on the right track. It reinforces the effectiveness of your approach and helps you feel confident in your abilities, which is crucial when you are documenting something as important as a case study.

Types of Feedback to Seek

When gathering feedback, it is important to seek input from various sources. Each type of feedback offers a different lens to evaluate your case study and combining them can give you a well-rounded view of your work.

Client Feedback

Clients are the heart of any case study, and their perspective is invaluable. After completing their treatment or the assessment portion of your case study, ask them how they felt throughout the process. Did they feel comfortable with the communication and treatment plan? Did they feel involved in the decision-making process? Their input can help refine how you approach client engagement and ensure that your treatment techniques are having the desired effect.

Peer Review

Feedback from fellow massage therapists, colleagues, or mentors can help you assess the technical aspects of your case study. Did you choose the right treatment techniques? Is the structure of your case study sound? Did you miss anything critical? Peer review is necessary to ensure that your findings meet professional standards and that your methodology is solid.

Mentor or Expert Feedback

If possible, seek feedback from someone with more experience in conducting case studies or someone with expertise in the area you are studying. Obtaining an expert's feedback can help you to elevate the quality of your case study and ensure that it aligns with best practices within the profession.

Self-Reflection

Do not forget to take a moment to review your own work critically. Ask yourself questions like: Did I address all the key points? Is my analysis thorough? How well did I communicate my findings? Self-reflection gives you a chance to assess your growth and pinpoint areas for improvement without outside influence.

Incorporate Feedback into Your Case Study

Once you have gathered feedback, it is time to adjust your case study.

Here is how you can effectively incorporate that input into your case study process:

Be Open to Criticism

Constructive criticism might not always feel great in the moment, but it is an opportunity to grow. Be open to suggestions and avoid taking feedback personally. Instead, view it as a tool that helps you become better at what you do. Remember, every piece of feedback is an opportunity for improvement!

Look for Patterns

If multiple people point out the same issue, it is a sign that this is an area that needs your attention. Look for recurring themes in the feedback and address these first. Whether it is related to clarity, treatment protocols, or data collection, making these adjustments will enhance the overall quality of your case study.

Adjust Based on Client and Peer Input

For example, if a client shares that they did not fully understand the treatment plan or felt confused about certain aspects of the process, you should consider revising how you communicate those details. Similarly, if a peer mentions that you could have expanded on certain treatment outcomes, take the time to add more context or data to support your conclusions.

Do not Overcorrect

While it is important to make improvements, avoid overcorrecting based on feedback. Too much tweaking can make your case study lose its original focus or cause you to deviate too far from your initial goals. Focus on enhancing clarity and depth, rather than radically changing the approach unless absolutely necessary.

Use Feedback to Evolve Your Practice

Feedback is not just about improving your case study—it is also a chance to evolve your practice. As you incorporate feedback, pay attention to how your overall approach to client care and case study methodology begins to shift. You might notice new techniques, better ways to communicate, or more efficient ways to structure your future case studies.

Continuous Improvement

Incorporating feedback is a continual process. After completing one case study, take the lessons learned and apply them to the next one. Each time you go through the process, you will find areas for refinement, which will ultimately make your approach more effective and streamlined.

Evolving Treatment Plans

If feedback from peers or clients reveals that certain treatment approaches were more effective than others, use that knowledge to update your future treatment protocols. Consider adding new techniques or adjusting how you approach certain conditions based on what worked well in the case study.

Contributing to the Community

As you incorporate feedback into your own practice, you can also use it to help others. Whether it is through mentoring, writing articles, or sharing your case study insights at conferences, when you share what you have learned from feedback it helps elevate the profession as a whole.

Incorporating feedback is one of the most powerful ways to refine your case studies and your practice. By seeking input from clients, peers, and mentors, and then using that feedback to improve your work, you are setting yourself up for ongoing success. Remember, feedback is a tool for growth, and when embraced with an open mind, it can take your case studies—and your practice—to the next level.

Refine and Improve

Feedback is not criticism—it is a gift.

1. **Find a Feedback Buddy:** Choose a trusted colleague or mentor to review your draft report.
2. **Ask Specific Questions:** Write down 2–3 focused questions for them (e.g., "Is my conclusion clear?" "Are my visuals helpful?").
3. **Reflect on Feedback:** After you receive feedback, write down one thing you will change and one thing you will keep the same.

How did the feedback improve your case study?

Page left intentionally blank for your notes

Advanced Case Study Techniques

Longitudinal Case Studies

When it comes to case studies, many professionals might find themselves focusing on short-term assessments, which are useful, but there is a whole other level of insight that comes from looking at the long-term effects of treatment. That is where longitudinal studies come into play. These types of studies follow clients or patients over an extended period to observe the long-term outcomes and trends.

Let's dive into the world of longitudinal studies, where the focus is on tracking progress over time and how this can be a game-changer for both your practice and the profession as a whole.

What is a Longitudinal Study?

At its core, a longitudinal study is one that tracks a subject (or subjects) over a longer period, often ranging from months to even years. Rather than just capturing a snapshot of a single moment, longitudinal studies capture data and observations over time, allowing you to see how things evolve.

For example, if you are studying the effects of a particular massage therapy technique on chronic pain, a longitudinal study would involve measuring pain levels at multiple intervals over several months or years. This approach provides a more comprehensive picture of the treatment's long-term effectiveness.

Why Use Longitudinal Studies?

The true power of a longitudinal study lies in the insights it can provide about sustained changes over time. Unlike a short-term case study, which may show immediate results, a longitudinal study helps you understand whether those results are sustainable, how they develop, and if any new patterns emerge as time goes on.

Tracking Progress Over Time

Longitudinal studies allow you to track how clients' conditions evolve after treatment and how interventions lead to lasting changes. By measuring progress at regular intervals, you can determine if treatment plans are leading to sustained improvements or if you need to make modifications.

Revealing Trends

Sometimes, the full effect of a treatment takes time to show. Longitudinal studies help you identify patterns that might not be immediately obvious. For instance, you might find that a client experiences gradual improvement in flexibility over the course of six months, but only after continuous treatment rather than after a single session.

Understanding Long-Term Effects

Many interventions, especially in therapeutic practices, have effects that extend beyond the immediate results. A longitudinal study can reveal the long-term benefits or side effects of a treatment, helping you refine your approach and inform future practice.

Designing a Longitudinal Study

When it comes to designing a longitudinal study, the process can feel a bit more complex than short-term case studies. You will need to ensure that your study is structured to capture consistent, reliable data over time.

Set Clear Objectives

Just like with any case study, start by defining clear objectives for your longitudinal study. What do you want to track over time? Are you focused on symptom relief, treatment adherence, or overall health improvements? Having a focused goal will help you stay on track throughout the duration of the study.

Determine Your Data Points

Longitudinal studies often involve multiple data points over an extended period. You will need to decide how frequently you will measure outcomes. Will you collect data every week, month, or quarter? The key is to find a balance between gathering enough information to see trends, while not overwhelming yourself or your clients with too frequent measurements.

Choose the Right Tools

Tracking progress over time requires tools that allow you to collect consistent data. Whether it is pain scales, range-of-motion measurements, or self-reported questionnaires, make sure you choose reliable methods that you can consistently apply throughout the study.

Be Prepared for Setbacks

In a longitudinal study, it is common to encounter bumps along the road—clients may drop out, there could be missed appointments, or you might face other unexpected challenges. The key is to stay flexible and adapt as needed, ensuring that you are still collecting valuable data while remaining open to course correction.

Advantages of Longitudinal Studies

The beauty of longitudinal studies is that they give you a deeper, more nuanced understanding of the impact of your treatments.

By tracking long-term data, you will be able to make more informed decisions about treatment plans and strategies. If your study shows that certain techniques consistently lead to better long-term outcomes, you can make more targeted recommendations for your clients.

In the world of evidence-based practice, having a longitudinal study under your belt gives you solid data to back up your claims. It can serve as a solid foundation for recommending treatments to your clients or sharing your findings with the broader massage therapy community.

When you engage in long-term follow-up and tracking, clients can see that you are committed to their progress. This builds trust and strengthens the therapeutic relationship. Plus, they will appreciate that you are tracking their results to ensure their well-being is continuously prioritised.

Challenges of Longitudinal Studies

While the benefits are clear, conducting a longitudinal study does come with its fair share of challenges.

Longitudinal studies take time—sometimes a lot of it! Whether you are tracking progress over six months or several years, it requires sustained effort on your part to consistently collect and analyse data.

Clients may drop out of a longitudinal study for several reasons—busy schedules, changes in health status, or simply losing interest. It can be challenging to keep clients engaged over an extended period. Consider how you might encourage participation and maintain consistent communication to keep them involved.

The longer the study, the more data you will need to manage. Organising, storing, and analysing all that information can become overwhelming, especially if you are tracking multiple variables. Proper planning and the right tools will be crucial in ensuring you stay on top of the data.

Using Longitudinal Studies for Professional Growth

When done well, longitudinal studies can serve as an invaluable learning tool—not just for your clients, but for you as a professional. They give you insight into the long-term impact of your methods, which can help you refine your techniques and improve your practice.

The results of longitudinal studies can often be seen as more persuasive than short-term studies because they show consistent, sustained changes. They also give an opportunity for you to contribute valuable knowledge to the broader field of massage therapy, further establishing you as an expert in your area of practice.

Longitudinal studies may be a bit more complex than traditional case studies, but the insights they offer are invaluable. Tracking progress over time provides you with a deeper understanding of treatment outcomes, allowing you to make more informed decisions and deliver better care to your clients. With careful planning, consistent tracking, and an open mind, you can incorporate longitudinal studies into your practice and unlock new possibilities for growth and professional development.

Thinking Long-Term

These studies require patience, but they yield rich insights.

1. **Sketch a Long-Term Plan:** Write down how often you would revisit your client (for example, monthly, quarterly).

2. **Identify Long-Term Metrics:** What data points will you track over time? Write them down.
3. **Prepare Follow-Up Questions:** Draft 2–3 questions you will ask your client during each follow-up.

Reflection Prompt: *What excites you most about tracking long-term changes?*

Page left intentionally blank for your notes

Comparative Case Studies

Comparative case studies are a fascinating approach that can provide even deeper insights into how different treatments or techniques perform in various scenarios. If you have ever found yourself wondering, "How does this technique compare to that one?" or "Which treatment method yields the best results?", this is exactly where comparative case studies come into play.

So, what makes comparative case studies stand out?

What is a Comparative Case Study?

A comparative case study involves comparing two or more treatments, methods, or approaches to assess their effectiveness or outcomes. Instead of focusing on one client's progress, you are looking at multiple cases, each of which may involve different treatments, but with the same goal in mind. By drawing comparisons, you can highlight key differences and similarities between different methods, helping you and others understand what works best under various circumstances.

For example, let's say you are studying the impact of two different types of massage therapy techniques—deep tissue versus Swedish massage—on chronic back pain. By comparing client progress across both methods, you can evaluate the effectiveness of each technique and when one might be more appropriate than the other.

Why Use Comparative Case Studies?

Comparative case studies are powerful because they provide a broader perspective on treatment options and outcomes.

Sometimes, one treatment is not the right fit for every client. A comparative case study allows you to compare how different treatments work for similar issues, helping you understand which approaches are more effective under certain circumstances. For example, a client with a sports injury might respond better to a specific technique, while another client with chronic tension might benefit from something entirely different.

In your day-to-day practice, you will often face situations where you have to choose the right approach for a particular condition. A comparative case study allows you to draw on real data to guide your decisions. If you have seen success with one method over another, you can confidently use that information to support your treatment plans.

By comparing multiple treatment methods, you can also learn more about client preferences. For instance, one client might prefer the gentle approach of Swedish massage, while another might feel more benefit from a deep tissue session. Understanding these preferences, along with treatment effectiveness, helps you tailor your practice to meet each client's needs.

Designing a Comparative Case Study

Just like with any case study, designing a comparative case study requires thoughtful planning. Here is how you can set yourself up for success:

- **Define what you want to compare**. Is it the effectiveness of two techniques on pain relief? Are you comparing outcomes based on different treatment frequencies? By setting clear, measurable goals, you ensure that your study remains focused and relevant.
- **Decide which cases you want to compare.** Do you want to study the impact of different techniques on a single client or multiple clients? You can compare two or more clients, each receiving different treatments. For example, one client might get Swedish massage for their back pain, while another might receive deep tissue massage. Alternatively, you might compare the effectiveness of treatment A in multiple clients versus treatment B.

For a comparative case study, data collection is key. You will need to capture the same types of information for each client involved. This could be things like pain levels, range of motion, or quality of life scores. By ensuring that your data points are consistent across cases, you will be able to make valid comparisons.

Just like in any case study, monitoring progress is crucial. Track each client's progress throughout their treatment, whether it is on a weekly basis or at intervals that make sense for the case. Comparing results at different points in time will help you spot trends and differences between treatments.

Advantages of Comparative Case Studies

The beauty of comparative case studies lies in the insights they provide by looking at multiple approaches.

Comparative case studies can give you a clearer picture of which treatment works best for specific conditions. For instance, you might discover that deep tissue massage works better for clients with muscle stiffness, while Swedish massage is more effective for clients with stress-induced tension. By comparing, you can fine-tune your recommendations and improve client outcomes.

When you compare multiple treatments and demonstrate their effectiveness or shortcomings, you are building a body of evidence. This not only strengthens your credibility as a professional but also adds to the collective knowledge of the massage therapy community. If you ever decide to publish or present your findings, comparative case studies give you a solid foundation to stand on.

Clients often want to know why you are choosing one treatment over another. With a comparative case study, you can share real-life data about how different methods work in practice. This can help educate your clients and set realistic expectations about their treatment options. They will feel more confident when they understand the reasoning behind your decisions.

Challenges of Comparative Case Studies

Like any research method, comparative case studies come with some challenges.

Each client is different, so comparing treatment effectiveness can sometimes be tricky. Even with similar conditions, individual responses to treatment can vary. It is important to acknowledge these differences when drawing conclusions, because what works for one client may not work as well for another.

When comparing treatments, you are likely dealing with multiple variables that can affect outcomes—client age, previous injury history, lifestyle habits, and even stress levels. Balancing all these variables while trying to isolate the impact of the treatments themselves can be challenging. The more variables you introduce, the harder it becomes to pinpoint the exact reason one treatment might have worked better than the other.

A comparative case study requires thorough planning and data collection, which can be time-consuming. You will need to commit to regular follow-ups and track a variety of factors for each case. It can also be difficult to get consistent data across multiple clients or treatments, especially if you are working with a variety of techniques.

Applying Comparative Case Studies in Your Practice

While comparative case studies may take more effort to set up, they can be incredibly useful tools in refining your practice and contributing to the wider field of massage therapy.

By comparing different treatments and techniques, you will be able to fine-tune your approach and make more informed decisions about which methods to use in different situations. The insights you gain will make you more versatile as a therapist, able to adapt your approach based on what is likely to yield the best outcomes.

As with any case study, sharing your findings can help others in your field learn and grow. Whether it is through publishing your results, presenting at conferences, or simply discussing your findings with colleagues, comparative case studies contribute to the broader understanding of treatment efficacy and help elevate the profession as a whole.

Comparative case studies offer a unique way to examine different treatment methods, allowing you to compare outcomes and make informed decisions about the best approach for your clients. While they do come with some challenges, the rewards are well worth it. By gaining a deeper understanding of how different methods work, you can enhance your clinical skills, offer more personalised treatments, and contribute valuable knowledge to the massage therapy field.

Side-by-Side Stories:
Let's see what happens when you compare different cases.

1. **Choose a Comparison Point:** Write down one key aspect you would compare (e.g., two clients with similar conditions but different responses to treatment).

2. **List Similarities and Differences:** Create two quick lists—one for similarities, one for differences.
3. **Write a Mini-Analysis:** Write a short paragraph explaining one key insight from your comparison.

Reflection Prompt: *What surprised you most when comparing these cases?*

Page left intentionally blank for your notes

Collaborative Case Studies

This section discusses **collaborative case studies**—a wonderful approach where professionals from different backgrounds work together to analyse and solve a complex issue. In the world of massage therapy, this is an exciting opportunity to connect with others, whether they are from within your field or from related disciplines, like physiotherapists, occupational therapists, or even doctors. It is about bringing together expertise to enhance treatment outcomes and deepen your understanding of a client's needs.

What is a Collaborative Case Study?

A **collaborative case study** is when multiple professionals come together to address a specific client's condition or treatment. Each professional brings their unique knowledge, skill set, and perspective to the table, creating a multidisciplinary approach to analysing and treating the client. This can lead to a more comprehensive understanding of the case and potentially better outcomes for the client.

For example, you might work alongside a physiotherapist to assess how your massage therapy techniques could complement their rehabilitation exercises. Or, if you are treating a client with chronic pain, collaborating with an occupational therapist could provide valuable insights into ergonomics and functional movement.

Why Use Collaborative Case Studies?

Working alongside other healthcare professionals opens you up to different approaches and new techniques that you may not have considered before. You might discover more effective ways of addressing client issues or gain insights into areas of your practice that you may not be fully aware of. For instance, a physiotherapist might show you a specific exercise that complements your massage therapy and accelerates recovery.

When you collaborate with others, you can create a more well-rounded and holistic treatment plan for your clients. If you are treating a client for pain relief, your massage techniques combined with a chiropractor's alignment adjustments or a nutritionist's advice about anti-inflammatory foods can address the issue from multiple angles, enhancing the overall treatment.

The real winner here is your client. When they see that a group of professionals is collaborating with their best interests at heart, it increases their confidence in the treatment. A collaborative approach means that clients receive a more comprehensive treatment plan that considers different facets of their health, potentially leading to better results in less time.

Designing a Collaborative Case Study

As with any case study, designing a collaborative case study takes planning because you must coordinate with other professionals, which means more moving parts.

The key to a successful collaborative case study is clear communication. Start by outlining who is involved and what each professional's role will be. Is your focus primarily on massage therapy, or are you working together on a treatment plan? Define what each professional will bring to the table and set clear objectives for the study.

For instance, you might take the lead in assessing the client's muscle tension and pain management, while a physiotherapist could focus on strengthening exercises. The more defined your roles are, the more smoothly the collaboration will run.

It is essential that everyone on the team agrees on the goals and outcomes you are hoping to achieve. Are you aiming to reduce a client's pain by 50 percent within a certain timeframe? Do you want to see improvements in mobility or function? Everyone needs to be on the same page about what success looks like for the client.

When it comes to gathering data for a collaborative case study, you are looking at a lot of shared information. Each professional will be collecting data from their own perspective—pain assessments, range of motion measurements, exercise progress, etc. Make sure you have an agreed-upon system for recording and sharing this data so that everyone involved can stay informed and contribute to the case study's analysis.

Advantages of Collaborative Case Studies

There are so many great reasons to take the collaborative route.

Collaboration lets you offer a treatment plan that integrates various approaches. By pooling expertise, you are providing your client with a treatment that looks at all the factors contributing to their issue, from muscle tension to posture, lifestyle, nutrition, and more. A multidisciplinary plan addresses the problem from all angles, which often leads to faster and more lasting results.

By collaborating with other professionals, you are not just helping your clients—you are also learning and growing. This is a fantastic way to expand your own professional network and deepen your understanding of other therapeutic disciplines. Plus, it can open doors for future collaborations and referrals, which can grow your practice.

When you collaborate with well-respected professionals, it enhances your own credibility. Clients will see that you are open to working with others to provide the best possible care. And, when you are willing to share the spotlight and respect the expertise of other professionals, it helps build trust and encourages a more holistic view of care.

Challenges of Collaborative Case Studies

As much as collaborative case studies have their benefits, they can also come with a few challenges.

When you are working with multiple people, especially from different disciplines, miscommunication can happen. This is why it is critical to have clear expectations, defined roles, and open lines of communication from the start. Regular check-ins and clear documentation help ensure that everyone is on the same page and that nothing is overlooked.

Each professional in the collaborative case study may have their own treatment philosophy and approach. This can sometimes lead to disagreements or differences of opinion on the best course of action for the client. The key to overcoming this is open dialogue and respecting the unique contributions of each professional. Remember, you are all working toward the same goal—improving the client's well-being.

Coordinating schedules can be tricky when multiple professionals are involved. You will need to find a time that works for everyone to meet and discuss the case study, review the client's progress, and make decisions. It is important to build flexibility into your approach and keep the lines of communication open to avoid any scheduling frustrations.

Applying Collaborative Case Studies in Your Practice

Now that you know how to design and execute a collaborative case study, it is time to start applying the insights you gain.

By taking a more holistic, multidisciplinary approach, you can significantly improve client outcomes. You will be able to see the treatment from multiple angles and address a range of factors contributing to the client's condition. This could lead to a more tailored and effective treatment plan, setting you apart as a thorough and innovative practitioner.

If you work on a collaborative case study, use it as an opportunity to share your results with others in your profession. Whether you present it at a conference, write a paper, or simply discuss the findings with your colleagues, sharing your insights helps to broaden the knowledge base in the field and fosters a community of learning.

Working on a collaborative case study will help you to build relationships with other professionals. It is a chance for you to expand your professional network and create connections that can lead to future collaborations. This will not only benefit your practice but also your clients, who will appreciate the well-rounded, team-oriented approach to their care.

Collaborative case studies offer a fantastic opportunity to elevate the level of care you can provide by combining the knowledge and expertise of multiple professionals. While they do come with their own set of challenges, the benefits—ranging from more comprehensive treatment plans to professional development—make it well worth the effort. By applying these insights, you can offer clients the best possible care, all while growing your practice and contributing to a greater understanding of effective treatment strategies.

Teamwork Makes the Dream Work

Collaboration can bring fresh perspectives and deeper insights.

1. **Find a Collaborator:** Think of one colleague who might be interested in working on a case study with you.

2. **Outline Roles:** Write down who will oversee which tasks (for example, assessments, data collection, report writing).
3. **Set a Communication Plan:** Decide how often you will check in with your collaborator and how you will share updates.

Reflection Prompt: *What strengths does your collaborator bring to the table?*

Page left intentionally blank for your notes

Future Trends in Case Studies

As the world of massage therapy continues to evolve, so too does the practice of conducting and using case studies. In the future, we can expect several exciting trends that will shape the way we approach case studies, from technology-driven tools to shifts in how we collect and analyse data. This section looks at some of the trends that may influence case studies in the years to come.

Increased Use of Technology

The future of case studies in massage therapy is heavily influenced by technology. We are already seeing how digital tools can help streamline the process, but as technology advances, the possibilities for case studies are expanding. From virtual assessments to data analysis software, we can expect technology to play an even bigger role in making case studies more efficient and accurate.

Virtual and Remote Assessments

Remote consultations and virtual assessments could become more common, particularly with the rise of telehealth. As long as the client is comfortable and the assessment is appropriate for remote work, conducting initial assessments or follow-ups through video calls could provide more flexibility and reach for massage therapists, which can make it easier to collaborate with clients regardless of location.

AI and Data Analytics

Artificial intelligence and machine learning could become integral tools for analysing case study data. These technologies could help identify patterns, trends, and correlations in data that might not at first be obvious. For example, AI could assist in tracking a client's progress over time by analysing pain levels, mobility improvements, or even subjective feedback, offering insights that help guide treatment plans.

Integration of Wearable Technology

Wearable devices, such as fitness trackers and smartwatches, are currently used for health and wellness, but their use in case studies could become more prevalent. These devices can track a client's movement, sleep patterns, heart rate, and other important health metrics that could help to assess progress or even identify areas for improvement during treatment.

Real-Time Data Collection

Wearable technology could provide real-time data that enhances case study observations. For example, a client might wear a device that tracks their posture or muscle activity during daily tasks, giving the therapist real-time feedback on how well a treatment plan is working. This data can then be analysed to make quick adjustments, ensuring that the treatment remains effective.

Improved Client Monitoring

Wearables could also be used to monitor clients' progress between sessions. This allows therapists to see how their clients are responding to treatment and whether adjustments are necessary without having to wait until the next in-person session. This also empowers clients to take a more active role in tracking their progress.

Personalised and Holistic Approaches

The future of case studies may see a greater emphasis on personalised care. As we move toward a more holistic understanding of health, case studies may focus less on isolated symptoms and more on the entire person. This means not only looking at physical factors but considering mental, emotional, and environmental influences on health as well.

Multi-Disciplinary Collaboration

Collaborative case studies, as we have discussed, are likely to become more prevalent, particularly as the healthcare field continues to embrace a more interdisciplinary approach. By collaborating closely with professionals from various fields—such as nutritionists, physiotherapists, and even psychologists—massage therapists can create more comprehensive, client-focused treatment plans.

Personalised Treatment Plans

Case studies in the future may involve a deeper dive into clients' individual histories, preferences, and lifestyles to create highly tailored treatment plans. Advances in data analytics could help identify unique needs based on a client's personal background, genetics, and lifestyle factors. This would enable massage therapists to craft treatment strategies that are more customised and effective for everyone.

Shift Toward Preventative Care

There is a growing emphasis on prevention over treatment in healthcare, and this is likely to influence case studies as well. Rather than only focusing on fixing existing issues, future case studies may also focus on preventing problems before they occur.

Proactive Monitoring and Risk Assessment

Instead of waiting for a client to experience pain or injury, therapists could use case studies to assess potential risks and implement preventative measures. This could involve monitoring posture, movement patterns, and lifestyle factors before problems arise, allowing therapists to intervene earlier and help clients avoid injuries in the first place.

Long-Term Health Goals

Future case studies might place a greater emphasis on long-term wellness goals. Instead of simply addressing a client's immediate concerns, the study could look at ways to maintain and improve overall health over time, creating a more sustainable model of care.

Greater Emphasis on Client-Centered Outcomes

As the healthcare field continues to evolve, client-centered care will become even more integral to case studies. This approach ensures that clients are not just passive recipients of care but active participants in their own treatment journey. Future case studies will likely focus on a client's unique needs, preferences, and values, ensuring that they are central to the entire process.

Feedback-Driven Adjustments

In the future, case studies may increasingly incorporate client feedback at every stage of the process. Instead of solely relying on the therapist's observations, feedback from clients about their experiences, comfort levels, and any changes they notice will play a key role in shaping treatment plans. This helps ensure that the treatment plan is not only effective but also truly aligned with the client's needs.

Client Empowerment

Clients will be more involved in decision-making, setting goals, and tracking progress. This shift means that case studies will evolve into more collaborative efforts between the therapist and client. Expect to see case studies that reflect a partnership where both the therapist and the client share responsibility for the success of the treatment plan.

Increased Accessibility and Global Reach

As more people gain access to online platforms, case studies may become more widely accessible, allowing for a broader understanding and application of massage therapy techniques across different populations.

Virtual Case Studies

We may see an increase in virtual case studies, where massage therapists and other health professionals can collaborate and share their findings globally. This could help spread new treatment methods, share challenges and successes, and offer support to professionals in remote areas. The increased accessibility of information will lead to a more collaborative global community.

Online Learning and Case Study Sharing

The future of case studies may also see more therapists sharing their findings online, either through webinars, social media, or other online forums. This will allow massage therapists from diverse backgrounds to learn from each other, adapt successful strategies, and continuously improve their practice.

Improved Reporting Standards

As the professional community for massage therapists continues to grow, we may see more standardised approaches to case study reporting, which will help ensure that case studies are both rigorous and accessible to a wider audience.

Standardised Formats

In the future, case studies may follow more standardised templates that allow for easier comparison and assessment. This could involve more structured data collection methods, clearer reporting formats, and better integration of visual aids to make case studies easier to read and understand.

Open Access Journals and Databases

Free access journals and shared online platforms might become more common, giving practitioners the opportunity to access, contribute to, and learn from a global collection of case studies. This would enable massage therapists to easily explore research, discover new treatment approaches, and apply them to their own practice.

The future of case studies in massage therapy is incredibly exciting. With advances in technology, a shift toward holistic and preventative care, and greater collaboration between professionals, case studies may continue to evolve into a more personalised, effective, and accessible tool for improving client outcomes. By embracing these future trends, we can not only enhance our practice but also contribute to the ongoing growth and development of our profession.

Looking Ahead

The field is always evolving—Let's dream a little.

1. **Research One Emerging Trend:** Look into one innovative approach or tool being used in case studies (For example, AI data analysis, wearable technology).
2. **Brainstorm Applications:** Write down one way this trend could be used in your future case studies.
3. **Set a Learning Goal:** Identify one skill or resource you would like to explore further.

How can staying ahead of trends improve your practice?

Page left intentionally blank for your notes

Build Your Own Toolkit

Knowledge is power, and your toolkit is growing.

1. **Make a Reading List:** Write down 2–3 books, articles, or resources you want to explore further.
2. **Join a Community:** Find one online forum, Facebook group, or professional association focused on case studies.
3. **Commit to Continued Learning:** Write one action you will take in the next month to keep developing your skills.

What is one resource you already love and would recommend to others?

Page left intentionally blank for your notes

Additional Resources

As you dive deeper into the world of case studies, it is helpful to have a variety of resources to refer to. These resources can expand your knowledge, offer practical tools, and provide guidance as you continue to develop your case study skills. This section includes some key resources to support your journey.

Books

"Case Study Research in Practice" by Helen Simons

This book provides a comprehensive overview of the case study research methodology, covering the process from start to finish, and offering helpful advice for designing and conducting case studies in various fields.

"The Case Study Handbook: How to Read, Discuss, and Write Persuasively About Cases" by William Ellet

While this book is more business-focused, it offers great insight into how to read, analyse, and write about case studies, which can be applied to therapeutic settings.

"Massage Therapy: Principles and Practice" by Susan G. Salvo

A well-rounded book on the fundamentals of massage therapy, which also includes case study examples that may inspire you as you build your own.

“Clinical Reasoning in Massage Therapy" by Sandy Fritz

A comprehensive guide to massage therapy exams with insights on anatomy, client care, and assessment techniques.

"Massage Therapy: Integrating Research and Practice" by Trish Dryden

A detailed guide on critical thinking in clinical settings, useful for developing and analysing case studies.

"Medical Massage Care's Massage Exam Study Guide" by David Morin

Explores evidence-based practices in massage therapy and how to incorporate research into your treatments.

Research Journals

Journal of Bodywork and Movement Therapies

A valuable resource for research on various massage therapy techniques, including case studies that showcase real-life applications and outcomes.

International Journal of Therapeutic Massage and Bodywork

A journal dedicated to massage therapy, where you can find case studies and research articles that can provide context and examples for your own studies.

Journal of Clinical Massage and Bodywork

Offers clinical case studies and research articles that can provide insights into best practices for conducting massage therapy-related case studies.

Online Courses and Webinars

The Massage Therapy Foundation's Website

They offer various educational resources, including webinars and courses on conducting research and case studies. The foundation's focus is on improving the standards of massage therapy practice, making it an excellent resource for case study methodologies.

International Association of Massage Therapists (IAMT)

IAMT offers online resources, courses, and webinars focused on advancing the practice of massage therapy, including tips on how to incorporate case studies into your practice.

Coursera and edX

Platforms like these offer a wide range of online courses, including those that focus on research methodology, data analysis, and clinical study design, all of which can be beneficial for conducting thorough and impactful case studies.

Professional Organisations

Massage Therapy Associations

Most Massage Therapy Associations provide various resources for members, including research guidelines and access to a community of professionals who can provide feedback on case studies.

Australasian Lymphology Association (ALA)

As you work with case studies related to lymphatic health, the ALA offers specialised resources and support for lymphoedema professionals, including research and educational materials.

British Columbia Massage Therapy Association (BCMTA)

Another organisation offering resources, including guidelines and examples of research and case studies in the field of massage therapy.

Online Tools for Case Study Design

Google Scholar

A free and comprehensive resource for finding scholarly articles, research papers, and case studies across a range of topics. It is a great place to begin your research on any specific aspect of case study methodology.

Mendeley

A reference manager and academic social network that can help you organise your research, share case studies, and keep track of useful articles related to massage therapy case studies.

SurveyMonkey and Google Forms

If you need to gather data or feedback from clients or peers for your case studies, these platforms are great for creating and distributing surveys to collect detailed information.

Professional Development and Networking

Groups and Forums

Joining groups or professional forums focused on remedial massage therapy can connect you with others who are conducting or have conducted case studies. These communities can be invaluable for sharing experiences, getting feedback, and collaborating on research.

Annual Conferences and Workshops

Attending conferences like the **Massage and Myotherapy Australia Conference** or the **Australasian Lymphoedema Association Conference** can expose you to innovative research and case studies in your field. Many conferences also offer workshops or presentations that dive deep into case study methodologies.

Therapist Forums and Groups

Online therapist communities, like the **Massage Therapy Exchange** or specific groups for massage therapists, often discuss real-life case studies and share experiences, which can offer valuable insight.

Ethical Resources

National Institutes of Health (NIH) – Ethical Guidelines for Research

A great starting point to explore ethical standards in clinical research, which you can apply to your case studies to ensure compliance and integrity in your work.

The Ethical Guidelines for Health Researchers A comprehensive resource on ethics in healthcare research, including tips for confidentiality, informed consent, and handling sensitive data.

Data Analysis Software

Statistical Package for the Social Sciences (SPSS)

If you need to analyse large datasets from your case studies, SPSS is a great tool for statistical analysis. It helps with examining relationships between variables and identifying trends.

NVivo

NVivo is perfect for qualitative research and is useful if you are collecting and analysing narrative data from client interviews, observations, or journal entries. It helps you code and categorise responses to make sense of complex information.

Case Study Examples

Massage Therapy Case Studies: A Reference for Practitioners

A book or online database that shares various case study examples, offering both success stories and challenges to learn from. This can provide inspiration and structure as you develop your own case studies.

These resources can help you broaden your understanding of case study methodology, offer practical tools for gathering data, and provide ethical guidance. Keep exploring and engaging with these materials as you continue your journey into the world of case studies. The more you learn, the more confident you will feel in conducting your own, and the better equipped you will be to contribute to the field of massage therapy.

Templates

A structured guide for writing a comprehensive case study report

- **Title Page**: [Your Name], [Date], [Title of Case Study], [Professional Details]
- **Abstract**: Summary of the case (150-250 words)
- **Introduction**: Client background, context, and relevance of the study
- **Methodology**: Steps taken during assessment, treatments applied, and monitoring process
- **Results**: Data collected, observations, and visual aids (charts, photos)
- **Discussion/Conclusion**: Analysis of findings, key insights, recommendations
- **References**: APA-style citations for any external resources used
- **Appendices**: Photos, session notes, and extra documentation

Client Assessment Form

Include this on your form during the first session to document the client's baseline condition.

- **Client Details**: Name, Age, Contact Information
- **Medical History**: Relevant health background (injuries, surgeries, etc.)
- **Main Concerns**: Client's primary complaint
- **Observational Notes**: Posture, movement restrictions, pain levels
- **Consent Section**: A clear signature section for informed consent

Treatment Plan Template

Map out the treatment objectives, techniques, and track progress.

- **Treatment Goals**: Short- and long-term objectives
- **Planned Treatments**: Techniques (massage, cupping, etc.) and rationale
- **Session Log**: Date, method used, feedback from the client
- **Adjustments**: Any modifications in treatment due to progress or issues
- **Progress Notes**: Positive changes, ongoing concerns, next steps

Data Collection

For a systematic way to gather data throughout the case study include the following fields:

- **Measurement Dates**: Record each date that you collect data.
- **Quantitative Data**: Pain levels (scale 1-10), range of motion, and mobility tests
- **Qualitative Data**: Client feedback on pain, functionality, and overall wellness
- **Progress Charting**: Visual representation of improvements using graphs or tables

Photography Consent Form

ALWAYS obtain written client permission for using photographs and keep a copy for your records.

Key Sections of the consent form should include:

- **Why Photos are taken**: Explain the purpose for the photographs (for example, tracking progress, report presentation)
- **Where Photos will be used**: examples of uses include in the Case study report, conference presentation, etc.
- **Date and Client Signature**: Include space for a signature and date for legal consent.

Peer Feedback Form

Suggested Structure for obtaining constructive feedback from peers.

- **Strengths of Case Study**: What worked well in the study?
- **Suggestions for Improvement**: How can the report or study be enhanced?
- **Clarity of Goals and Results**: Are the objectives and conclusions clear?
- **Feedback on Presentation**: Was the case study effectively communicated?

About the Author

Andrea is an experienced massage therapist and educator specialising in advanced lymphatic management and remedial techniques. With a passion for empowering massage therapists to excel in their practice, she has created comprehensive courses and resources designed to deepen professional knowledge and enhance client care.

Throughout her career, Andrea has worked with a variety of clients, gaining firsthand experience in the complexities of treatment and rehabilitation. She is also a strong advocate for the role of massage therapists in healthcare, particularly in the recognition and integration of massage therapy in multidisciplinary treatments plans.

Andrea has presented at major conferences such as the Australasian Lymphoedema Association and Massage and Myotherapy Australia, and is committed to fostering collaboration, innovation, and peer review within the massage therapy community. She believes that sharing case studies and research is crucial for advancing the profession and improving outcomes for clients.

This book is a reflection of her years of practical experience and dedication to education. Building upon her popular online course, "Conducting Case Studies for Massage Therapists," Andrea offers a step-by-step guide to help therapists design, implement, and evaluate case studies effectively. Through examples, practical tips, and expert advice, Andrea provides invaluable insights to help both new and seasoned therapists develop their skills in conducting meaningful case studies that drive professional growth and client success.

When she is not writing or teaching, Andrea enjoys mentoring aspiring therapists and continuing to learn and grow in her field. Her mission is to support therapists in building their confidence, refining their skills, and contributing to the evolving landscape of massage therapy.

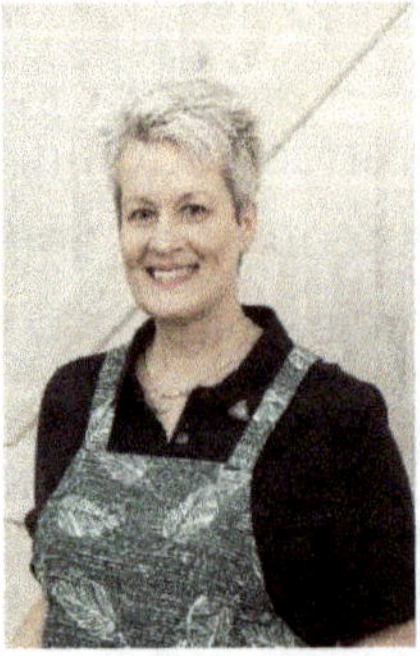

Other books by same author

Swollen with Swagger – Embracing Life with Lymphoedema

Lipoedema Unveiled – Navigating Life's Curves with Courage and Confidence (and a little bit of humour)

Imposter Syndrome BUSTED – From Self-Doubt to Confidence

These books and others are available on www.massagecpe.com.au

www.ingramcontent.com/pod-product-compliance
Lightning Source LLC
La Vergne TN
LVHW052243200926
848481LV00002B/261